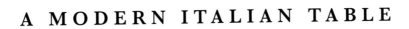

A MODERN ITALIAN TABLE

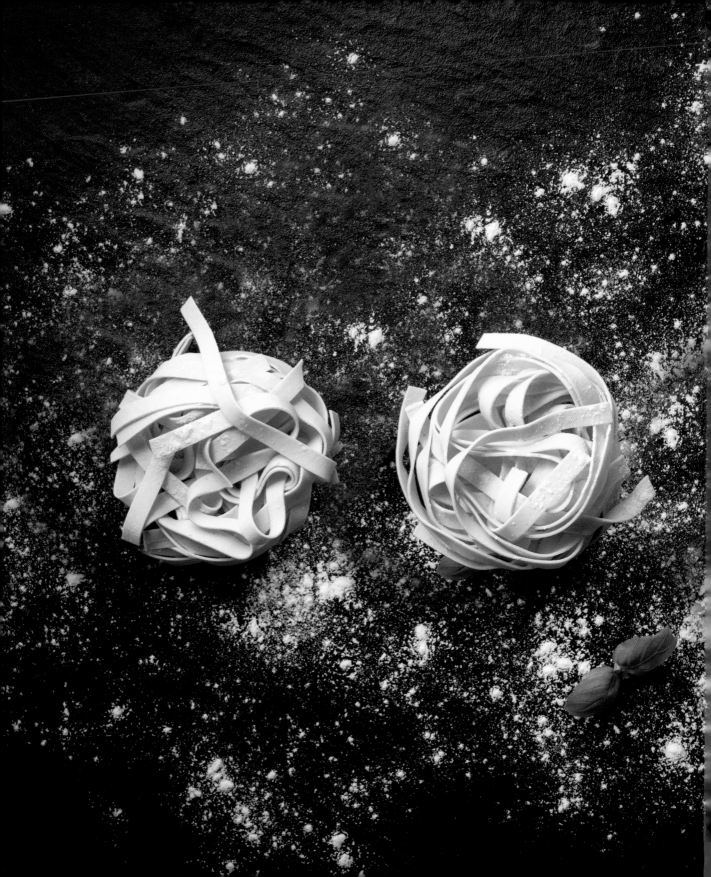

VERONICA LAVENIA

# A MODERN
# ITALIAN
# TABLE

NH
NEW
HOLLAND

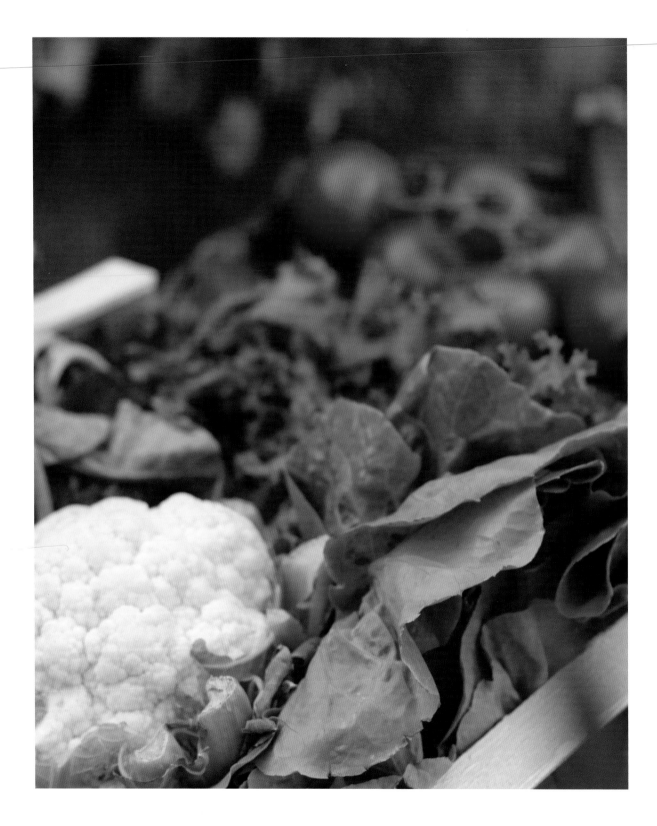

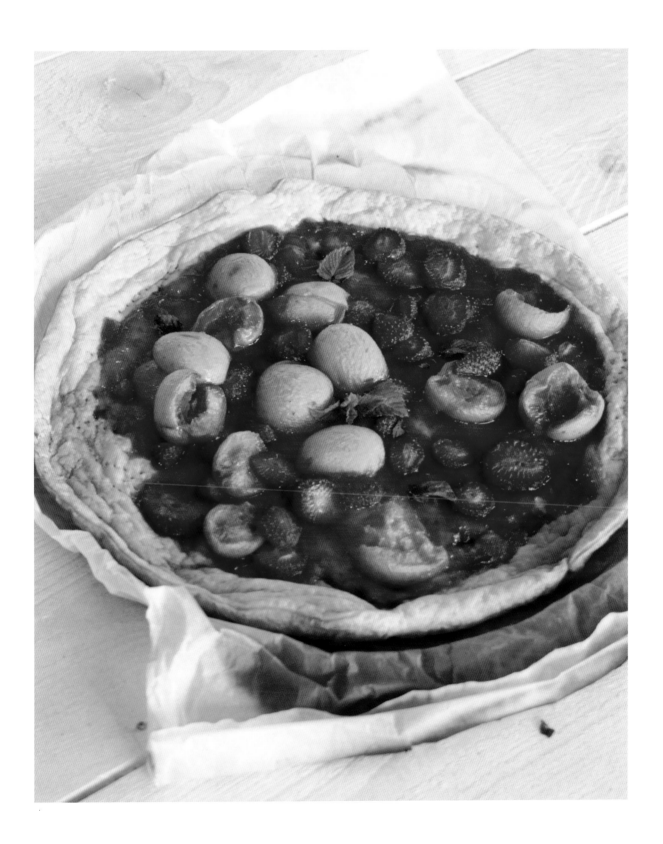

To people I love

Let your food be your medicine
and your medicine be your food.
*Hippocrates*

Simplicity is the ultimate sophistication.
*Leonardo Da Vinci*

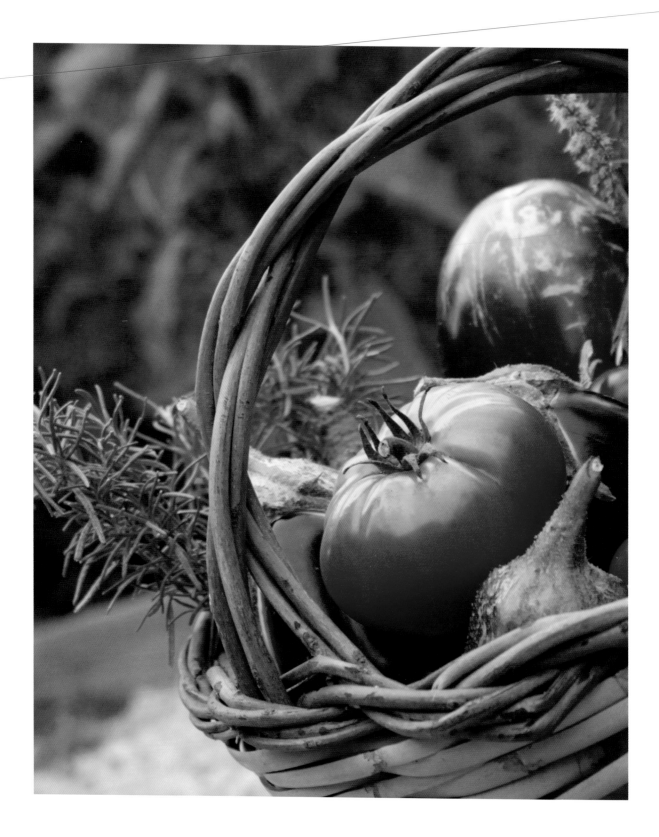

# CONTENTS

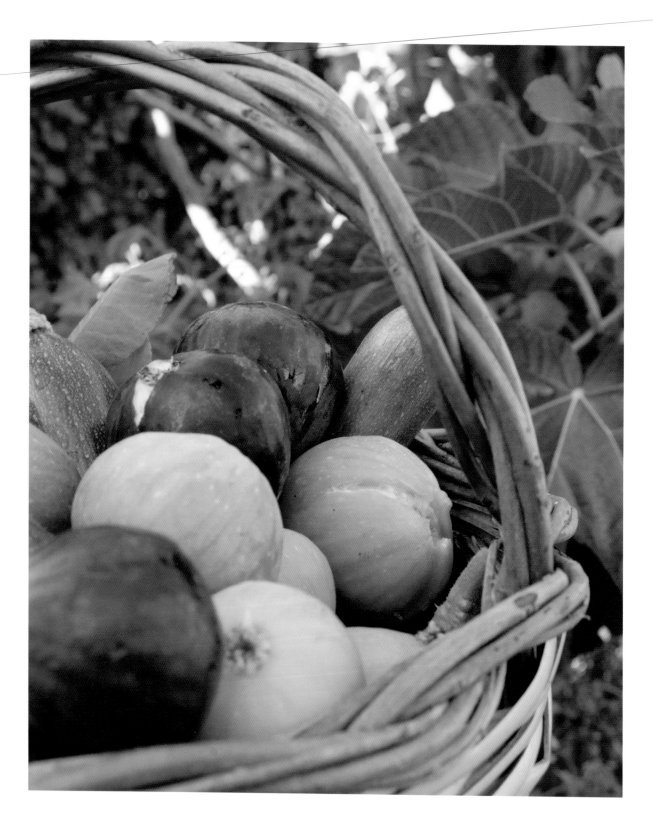

# INTRODUCTION

There is no need to eat a lot. The key is to eat well and with awareness. This is the teaching that was handed down to me by my parents since childhood and this is the philosophy of my books.

In an era in which food is demonized on several fronts and accused of being, more than a pleasure, the cause of many evils, Italian cuisine has not lost its essence, remaining unchanged in its fundamental basis and advancing with respect to the contemporary introducing ingredients from other cultures. The secret of the Italian tradition, on which I based my natural cuisine, is to evolve without losing its roots (or follow the culinary trends of the moment) but safeguarding the good and healthy food traditions of our ancient culinary heritage.

As with my previous works, freshness and seasonality are the basis for this book, as well as the high quality of the ingredients (organic and unrefined), which are readily available in supermarkets and specialty stores; Real, simple home cooking food that nourishes with taste and color. They are recipes I always eat at home with my family, some adapted according to my current tastes or contemporary needs. Italian (natural) cuisine is appreciated worldwide for its ease of implementation and for the few ingredients. Do not be surprised, therefore, if the steps of many of my recipes are as short as the ingredients. This is precisely the characteristic of true Italian cuisine. Less ingredients, fewer steps to execute and you will end up with a healthy and authentic dish.

The recipes are contemporary, uncomplicated and plant based (the majority Vegetarian and Vegan), using accessible ingredients to create amazing, natural dishes to enjoy every day.


Veronica

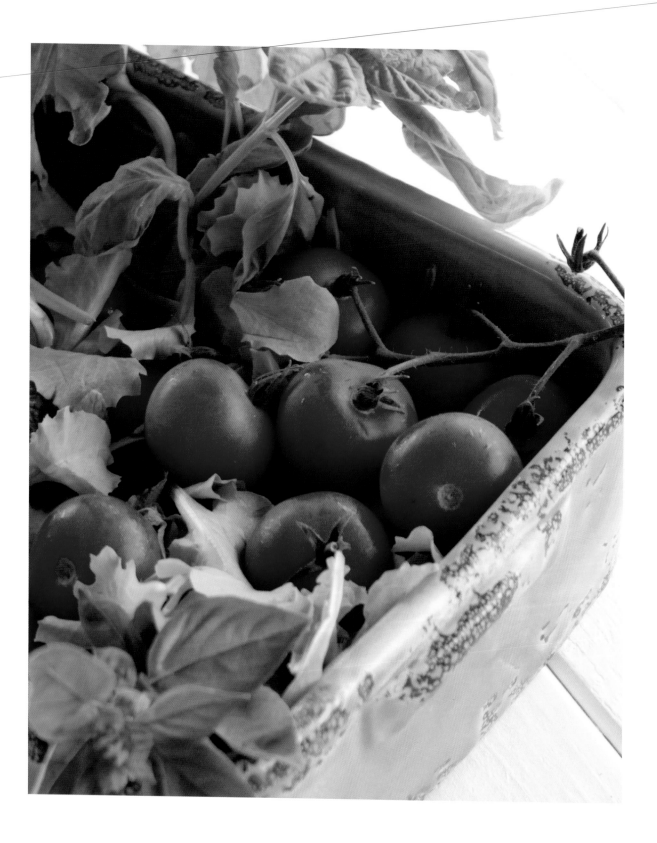

# MY NATURAL ITALIAN KITCHEN

In 'The Vegetarian Italian Kitchen' (and, before, in 'The Rustic Italian Bakery') I extensively wrote about what my pantry contains, giving useful tips for the consumption and preservation of vegetables and fruits, natural sweeteners, unrefined flours, oils and sea salt.

Vegetables and fruit are the basis of the Mediterranean Diet (UNESCO Intangible Heritage of Humanity), and along with cereals and legumes, are essential elements for a correct and healthy eating.

I find much of the seasonal vegetables from my family garden. For fruit and other organic vegetables, I prefer to stock up directly from farmers. In this way, I save money and, having established a relationship of trust with farmers, I am sure to buy good quality products. A good habit that I learned from my parents who, as a child, took me with them to shop not only in supermarkets but also on farms or in small food shops.

For those who live in the city, my suggestion is to buy, when possible, from farmers. If it is true that we are what we eat, taking the time to buy good, healthy, seasonal and unrefined food is a worthwhile investment whose benefits (in terms of costs and physical well-being) are immediate. This is true, especially in regards to certain foods such as eggs. I also buy them from farmers or from an organic shop near home. Free-range organic eggs are the result of happy hens, fed healthily. Eggs are a valuable food, rich in essential nutrients, especially for non-meat eaters. For this, it is advisable to buy only quality, certified eggs and always check the labels to make sure they are organic free range.

For oils, I only use extra virgin olive oil. In Italy, the choice is very wide. Extra virgin olive oils of Southern Italy have a very rich texture, a strong flavor and are particularly suited for savory recipes, while the Ligurian and Tuscan varieties have a more delicate taste and are also suitable for sweet preparations. I purchase a very special PDO extra virgin olive oil from a family company that has a long tradition in Sicily. I have another good reserve of extra virgin olive oil from some friends of mine who have a small farm on the slopes of Mount Etna (Sicily). From each trip to the various regions of Italy that produce oil, I always come back home with some new bottles of this precious nectar. In my family, we keep olive oil bottles like jewels. In fact, they are. As I wrote in 'The Vegetarian Italian Kitchen', the benefits of extra virgin olive oil are endless - it is the only oil extracted from a fruit, making it 100% natural. At the time of purchase, it is advisable to check the labels to certify the origin of the oil, the year of harvesting and extraction methods. When in doubt, leave it out.

The olive harvest (and the transformation in oil) has laborious and expensive processes. For this, a good quality extra virgin olive oil bottle has (or rather, must have) a high average cost.

For those who do not have the ease of finding a good extra virgin olive oil, the alternative is a good organic cold pressed sunflower oil.

Natural sweeteners are the healthiest choice you can make and they will give your recipes a naturally sweet flavour, and a lower glycemic index than white refined sugar. From raw honey (better if local), date nectar, coconut raw sugar or dark brown sugar, the choices are wide. Also dried fruit, like raisins or apricots, are great alternatives to white sugar on which the harmful effects on health have been widely debated for years.

For flours, I use unrefined whole grain flours. Sometimes, I use white flours but only from ancient grains such as Farro, Kamut or Sicilian ancient grains (such as Timilia or Tumminia - These flours are now available worldwide in the best Italian food shops). The so-called 'all purpose' and gluten free flours are over refined and subjected to chemical treatments which give a fake lightness and softness to the cakes.

The correct cooking of food is another key factor. An excellent ingredient may lose all its organoleptic characteristics and its health benefits if it is overcooked. I prefer to cook steam the vegetables (unless a recipe requires another type of cooking). Steaming keeps all the nutrients of vegetables intact.

A word about buying in supermarkets: Of course, in contemporary life, they are a useful reference point, but only if we buy with awareness. When I go to the supermarket I choose local products of small companies that spend little (or nothing, in some cases) in advertising and prefer to focus on the quality of their products and ingredients used. I always read the labels on the packaging. I avoid foodstuffs that exceed more than five ingredients and choose, whenever possible, to buy organic food because it is devoid of industry food additives, used to 'improve' the taste, smell and texture of food.

Another good habit is to ask. Although, by law, the labels should already define the ingredients, origin, nutritional values, date and place of production, including expiry date (and various certifications, different in each country), in cases where you have doubts, especially with regard to fresh good (fruits and vegetables, for example) do not hesitate to ask the retailer. If the answer does not convince you, or seems evasive, leave the product on the shelf. The market (but this applies to all) does not impose but proposes. The choice is ours. Many of us are always careful before buying a computer or a cell phone. The same attention should also be paid to the food we eat; our health depends on it.

The choice is not (only) between more or less good foods but between real and artificial food.

Eating healthy and affordable is not just a slogan for a niche of people. From this point of view, the Italian cuisine offers simple dishes, rich in taste, which capture everyone's attention.

This book continues the path of my earlier works, offering simple, natural recipes with tasty, readily available ingredients and uncomplicated cooking methods. The secret of Italian cuisine lies only in this and in the love we put in the food we cook.

If you are reading these pages, this philosophy of life is also yours. You just have to try and enjoy the pleasure of natural cooking, full of good and healthy food.

*Buon appetito!*

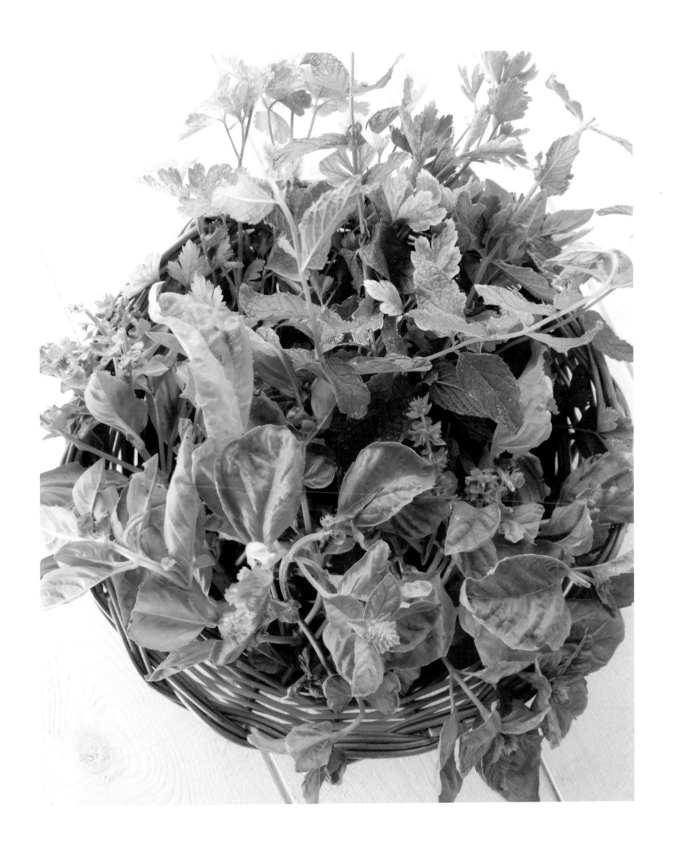

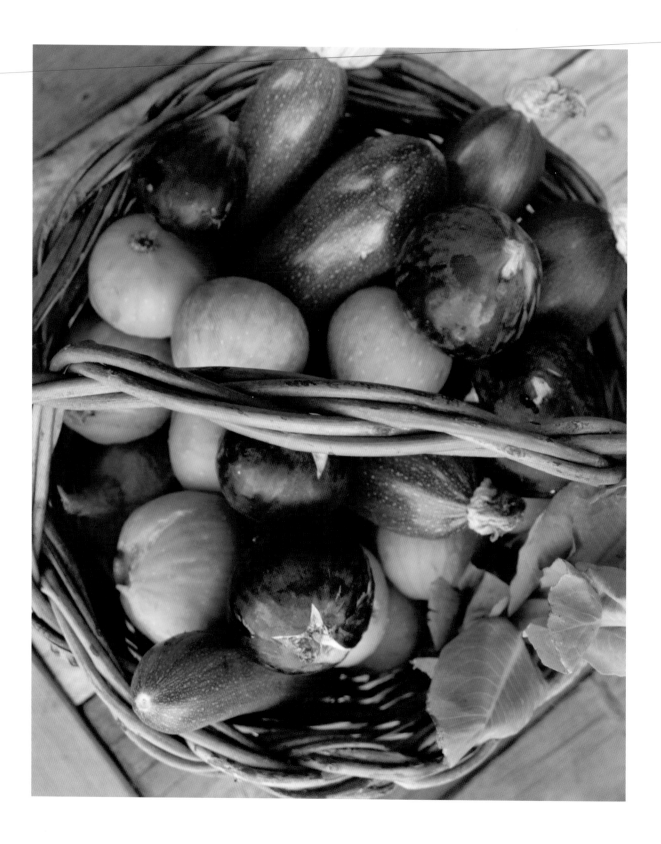

# BEAUTY AND HEALTH IN A SHELL

Among my favorite foods, dried fruit (with and without shell) are the leader of my table and it is to this precious food that I have decided to dedicate a few lines.

I learned to love them since the early days of my childhood. I remember many weekends spent in the forests around Mount Etna, in Sicily, collecting these valuable fruits.

Sicily is a land rich in almonds, pistachios, chestnuts, and hazelnuts. In other parts of southern Italy, such as the Amalfi Coast, you can enjoy small jewels of the territory as Sorrento walnuts or, a little farther on, the Giffoni hazelnuts, grown in the homonymous village, a few km from the Amalfi Coast. The hazelnuts of Piedmont are one of the culinary pearls of the North Italian territory, used, inter alia, also for the preparation of delicious hazelnuts spreadable creams.

Almost every country has places of dried fruit cultivation and that is why we must take advantage of these gifts of nature, rich in beneficial properties, often poorly understood.

I got to learn more about the properties of dried fruit over the years, thanks to a lot of reading on the subject, to farmers (which are for me always a source of much inspiration and knowledge) and a naturopath I met a few years ago.

Dried fruit appears in many of my recipes and is never a minor ingredient, even when it is used to decorate a dish.

Some of you may consider nuts, pistachios and hazelnuts unhealthy snacks because of their high calorie content. Instead, they are special ingredients for their valuable nutritional content of good fat, protein, vitamins, minerals and sugars.

They are allies of our inner and outer well-being, as high in those nutrients that nourish our body, also helping to keep our skin fresh and young (outer beauty, which some pursue relying on cosmetic surgery or expensive creams, first of all, go through healthy eating).

There are also medical researchers focused on the health benefits of nuts. Among the most recent studies on the topic, the New England Journal of Medicine published a study in 2013, and in 2014, the British Medical Journal. These, and other studies, have confirmed that the steady, moderate consumption of nuts helps to reduce cholesterol levels, inflammation, adiposity, helping to control sugar levels in the blood.

In addition to their proven physical benefits, the dried fruit is a topical ingredient that gives that extra touch to many recipes. For example, it can be used to make salads crispy and also enrich them with nutrients.

Hazelnuts are a source of vitamin C, and have a high percentage of potassium and vitamin E. Walnuts are rich in linoleic acid, are valuable in reducing bad cholesterol, and they contain vitamins A and B. Pistachios are source of iron and magnesium, copper, folic acid (and, like all nuts, they contain vitamin E). Almonds are a true anti-aging ingredient, rich in vitamin B2, phosphorus and calcium (found in the peel). Pine nuts, small but valuable, contain vitamins A, B, E, selenium, iodine and phosphorus. Chestnuts, rich in minerals such as phosphorus, magnesium and calcium, contain B vitamins and high in potassium.

With dried fruit (cashew, whole hazelnut and almonds, pistachios) you can also make a delicious, velvety butter. You just only have to soak the nuts for 6-8 hours (10-12 for almonds and hazelnut), and add 200 g (7 oz) dried fruit to your liking (cashews and almonds have a more neutral flavor that is also suitable for savory dishes). Drain and wash the dried fruit. Blend it with an immersion blender, adding a pinch of sea salt and 4-5 tbsp water until creamy. This healthy butter is perfect to be enjoyed spread on bread (alone or with jam) or for other preparations, (sweet and/or savory). It keeps in the refrigerator for 3-4 days.

A handful of dried fruit a day ensures health and well-being. Choose the local dried fruit in order to have better value for money and greater freshness. Regarding dried fruits without shells, it is better to buy organic raisins or apricots, making sure they are free from palm oil and chemical additives, which are often added to keep them soft.

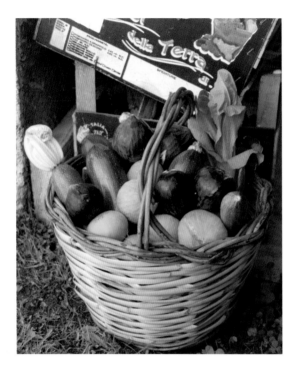 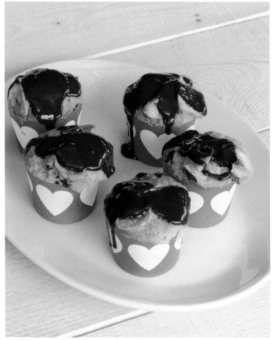

# AUTHOR'S NOTE

**CAKE TIN MEASUREMENTS:**
For cakes: 22 cm (8½ in) round tin (deep)
For pound-loaf cakes: 25 cm (10 in) (deep) loaf tin
For small cakes: 12-hole muffin tin or 12 cm (4½ in) round tin
For *crostatine* (little crostata/tarts) or small puff pastry cakes: mini molds (also with removable bottom)
 10 cm (4 in).

**CEREALS:**
The difference in cooking depends on the quality and type of cereal (if hulled or pearl barley, for example).
So, despite my cooking time suggestions, always check the instructions provided in the packaging you buy.

**EGGS:**
All eggs used in these recipes are organic free-range eggs, at room temperature.

**EXTRA VIRGIN OLIVE OIL:**
In Italy, there are no other types of olive oil, if not extra virgin. Often abroad, the extra virgin olive oil is only used to salads while, for cooking it is recommended to use 'regular olive oil'. For an Italian, it is hard to understand this distinction. In Italy, every oil that is not extra virgin has very low quality standards, mechanically extracted with solvents (Extra virgin olive oil differs from olive oil as it is extracted from the simple pressing of the olives with a maximum of 1% acidity. Olive oil, however, is made from a blend of refined and virgin olive oil with a maximum acidity of 1.5%). A good extra virgin olive oil is the best choice you can make for your health and to add flavor to your dishes.

How to choose a true extra virgin olive?
1. Be wary of cheap oils: An extra virgin olive oil sold at low cost it may not be true extra virgin. Better to apply directly to producers or specialty food stores selling exclusive products. A bottle of real olive oil has a higher cost but also has a longer life. So the value for money is profitable.
2. Read the labels: In Italy, there are very strict rules on food labels. They must indicate the brand, production process, place of production and product characteristics. Food labels must respect three fundamental characteristics: they must be clear, legible and indelible. As for extra virgin olive oil, for example, they must include the product name, expiration date and the origin of the oil.
3. Choose organic olive oil: Organic olive oil has a higher quality; it does not contain traces of pesticides and potentially harmful substances. The organic oil, preferably coming from small producers, does not contain the chemical correctors, often used by large industries to hide the acidity.
4. Choose PDO (DOP) and IPO (IOP) extra virgin olive oil: these are legally protected trademarks that defend the oil from counterfeits.

**FLOURS:**

As indicated, in this book I have only used unrefined flours. If you use white refined flours or white sugar, the amount of liquid and the final result change, as will the texture.

**FRUIT AND VEGETABLES:**

All fruit and vegetables used in these recipes are organic. Remove the peel if they are not.

**ORGANIC OR NATURAL BAKING POWDER:**

It should be aluminium free, and you should not use dry chemical baking powdes. Natural baking powder is available in the best supermarkets and organic food stores.

**PASTA:**

The cooking times are for the true Italian pasta, made with durum wheat flour or whole meal flours.
In Italy, by law, pasta is made only with durum wheat flour and not with soft flour (the same difference between a real pearl and stone). Pasta made with common flour (less expensive than semolina) leaves the water opaque (or white, in the worst cases) and not clear, as it should be. It also has a rubbery texture, no nutrition, is not easily digestible, often causing bloating in the stomach. Italian pasta must be cooked *al dente* (to the tooth). The standard portion in Italy, and the size recommended on Italian packages, is 80 g (3 oz).

**SWEETENERS:**

All unrefined organic sweeteners used in this book (raw honey; whole dates nectar/syrup; raw coconut sugar; raw brown sugar) are available in the best supermarkets and/or organic healthy food stores. Although they have a much lower glycemic index than white sugar, they are still sugar, even if natural. So, I suggest you follow the recommended doses, educating the palate to the less sweet flavors.

**TOFU:**

It is the basis of the Japanese diet, often considered among the healthiest of diets, just like the Mediterranean Diet (the Italians and Japanese are among the longest-lived people in the world).
Despite this, it is often at the center of controversial debates. This is because, outside of Japan, the soya beans, from which tofu is made, often come from genetically modified crops. Moreover, given the increase in demand, it is possible that the big food companies find cheaper ways of producing it. So, how to use this food considered beneficial in the Asian diet? The only way is to read the manufacturer's label. I buy organic non GM- tofu, with soya cultivated in Italy and I eat it no more than once a week. I usually find this kind of tofu also in traditional supermarkets.

**UNIT OF MEASURE:**

All measurements throughout this book are in grams, scientifically the most correct and used around the world (with the equivalent in ounces also provided). Measuring in ounces can be subject to changes in the various English-speaking countries. A digital grams-ounces scale is the best purchase that you can make.

**The recipes are described as follows:**

**DF- Dairy free**                    **VEG- Vegetarian**
**EG- Eggs free**                     **V- Vegan**
**GF: Gluten free**

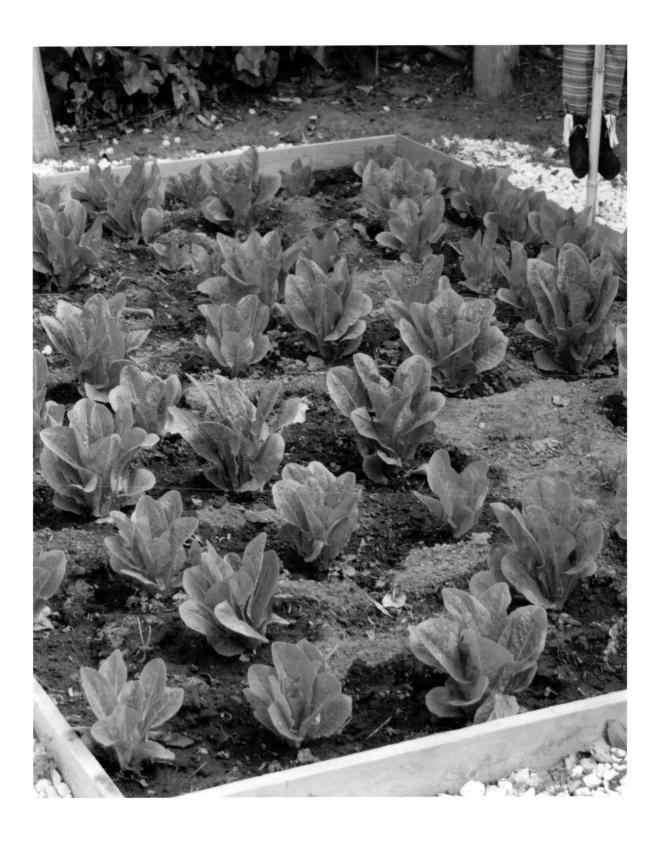

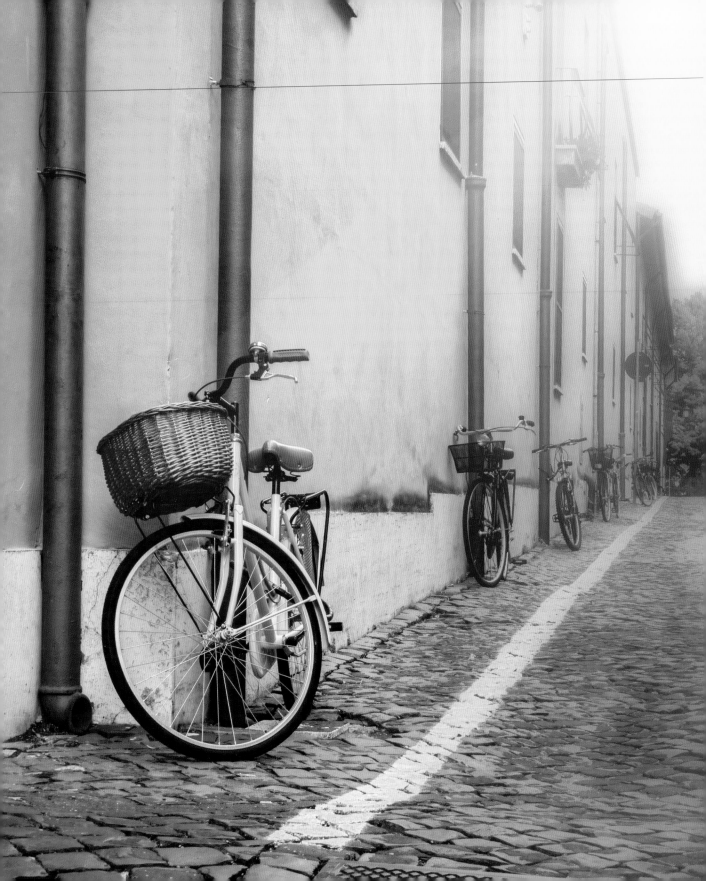

# SWEET AWAKENINGS

Breakfast is one of the most important meals of the day, the one that, during the week, we often devote little time to.

A nutritious and tasty breakfast is a very pleasant ritual, especially if made at home and shared with people we love.

In Italy, breakfast (which is not only "*Cornetto* and *Cappuccino*") has a very important value, even at a time when everyone seems to rush from the earliest hours of the morning. Homemade crostatas, biscuits (cookies) and cakes (in Italy, breakfast is strictly sweet) are a ritual that grandmothers and mothers trying to carry on.

My breakfast is simple but very tasty. As soon as I get up, I drink a glass of water with the juice of a lemon to purify and alkalize the body. Meanwhile, I set the table with care, just as I would do for lunch.

Usually, my breakfast table consists of some basic food stuffs such as rice milk (which I alternate, sometimes, with good organic goat's milk), brown rice cakes, raw honey and date nectar (and in summer, homemade jam and smoothies). I also believe it is important from early morning to reward yourself with homemade bakery items to alternate with the basic foods, such as cakes, cookies and tarts, all made with unrefined ingredients and white sugar. Unrefined cereals and flours provide the right energy and natural sweeteners, helping the palate become accustomed to more natural flavours, while controlling blood sugar spikes (but this does not mean you can abuse the consumption of natural sweeteners). A rich, healthy breakfast gives the right amount of energy to face the day and allows you to arrive at lunchtime without excessive hunger.

The recipes in this section are inspired by what I love to eat at breakfast (and even when I feel like a gourmet break). Very simple, natural recipes to enjoy alone or with friends for a breakfast rich in taste.

*This rustic apple cake has all the taste of organic apples in season. Be careful not to be seduced by the shiny, perfect apples that you find on most supermarket shelves. Demand the most for your health. Go in search of real, organic fruit, maybe less attractive at first glance, but still juicy.*

*The little things make the difference. The lightness of the rice yoghurt and mild olive oil give the dough a softness and smoothness. Wholemeal (whole-wheat) farro and almond flours, rich in nutrients, enhance the flavour of a timeless classic, which lends itself to many tasty but healthy variations.*

# APPLE CAKE

(TORTA DI MELE)

V

*Serves 4-6*

## INGREDIENTS

- 3 apples
- juice of 1 lemon
- 3 tablespoons rice-milk yoghurt
- 50 ml (1³/₄ fl oz) mild extra virgin olive oil (or 75 ml/3 fl oz cold-pressed
- organic sunflower oil)
- 60 g (2¹/₄ oz) raw coconut sugar
- 200 g (7 oz) wholemeal (wholewheat) farro

- flour, sifted (see note)
- 100 g (3¹/₂ oz) almond flour, sifted
- 15 g (¹/₂ oz) organic baking powder
- 1 teaspoon organic bourbon vanilla powder
- 100 ml (3¹/₂ fl oz) rice milk
- pinch of sea salt
- pinch of ground cinnamon
- 2 tablespoons slivered almonds

## METHOD

Preheat the oven to 180°C (350°F/Gas 4). Lightly grease and line a loaf (bar) tin with baking paper. Roughly chop the apples, drizzle with the lemon juice and set aside.

In a bowl, with the help of an electric mixer, whisk the rice-milk yoghurt, olive oil and coconut sugar until frothy. Add the sifted flours with the baking powder, vanilla, rice milk and salt and knead the ingredients until combined.

Pour the batter into the tin and add the apples on top. Bake for 35–40 minutes, or until lightly golden and a skewer inserted into the centre comes out clean.

Cool in the tin for a few minutes, then top with a sprinkling of cinnamon and sliced almonds. Lift out carefully onto a wire rack to cool completely.

*Note: Farro flour is made up of three wheat species: spelt, emmer and einkorn. It is sold dried in health food stores and specialty food stores.*

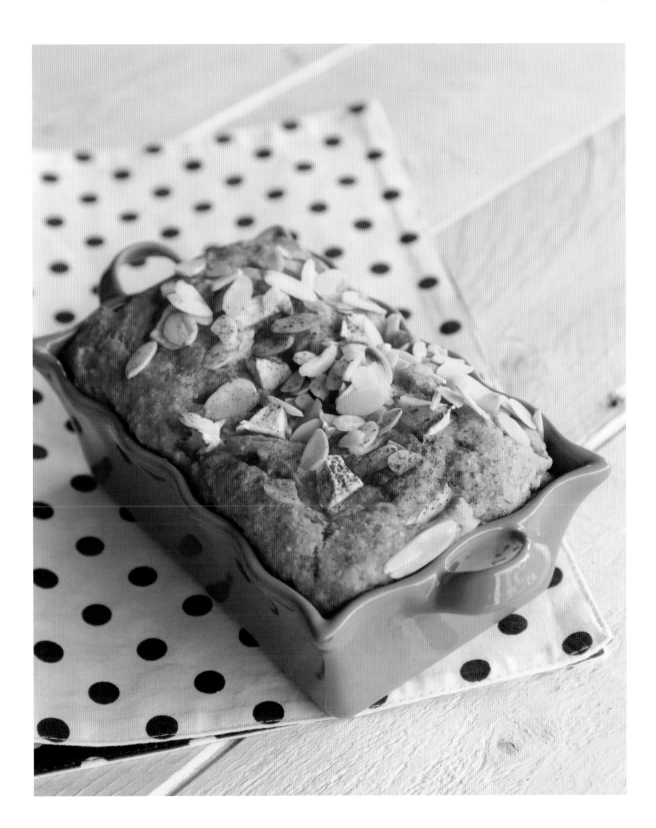

*This is a natural, tasty and easy raw pastry to make—rich in nutrients and energy. You can also add (or alternate) pistachio and walnuts.*

*The egg-free custard is the perfect match for these gluten and dairy-free tartlets and is also ideal to enjoy with seasonal fruit.*

# RED APPLE TARTS WITH EGG-FREE CUSTARD

(CROSTATINE DI MELE ROSSE CON FARCITURA DI CREMA SENZA UOVA)

DF-GF-VEG

*Serves 4*

## INGREDIENTS

### Pastry
· 100 g (3½ oz) almond flour
· 100 g (3½ oz) toasted hazelnut flour
· 50 g (1¾ oz) Medjoul dates
· 1 tablespoon raw honey

### Filling
· 3 tablespoons raw honey

· 60 g (2¼ oz) brown rice flour
· 60 g (2¼ oz) cornflour (cornstarch)
· 1 teaspoon organic vanilla bourbon powder
· 200 ml (7 fl oz) rice milk
· 1 orange zest
· 4 small red apples
· juice of 1 lemon

## METHOD
Preheat the oven to 180°C (350°F/Gas 4). Grease six round, fluted, loose-based flan tins.

### For the pastry:
Using a food processor or blender, combine the almond and hazelnut flour with the dates and honey. Place the mixture into the tart tins and refrigerate for about 15 minutes. Place in the oven to bake for 10 minutes, or until lightly golden.

### For the filling:
Combine the honey, flour and vanilla with 50 ml (1¾ fl oz) of the cold rice milk. Heat the remaining milk in a saucepan over medium heat and add the honey, flour, vanilla and 50 ml (1¾ fl oz) cold rice milk. Stir until the cream is thick. Add the orange zest. Leave to cool at room temperature, then put the cream in the fridge for 30 minutes.
Pour the cream over each tartlet. Cut the apples into wedges or cubes, according to liking, and place on top of the tartlets.

*Bananas are widely used in natural cuisine, not only because their sweetness makes cakes and cookies particularly tasty but also because they are a great thickener and make excellent egg substitutes. Not all bananas are the same and their choice is important to ensure that you get a healthy and quality product. Fairtrade bananas (available in most supermarkets or organic shops) are recommended because they provide a certificate product for the protection of the consumer and of the entire production chain.*

*Moist and soft, this cake has a unique aroma and is perfect to be enjoyed a few days after its preparation.*

# BANANA LOAF CAKE

## (TORTA DI BANANE)

EF- DF-VEG

### *Serves 6–8*

**INGREDIENTS**

- 250 g (9 oz) brown rice flour, sifted
- 50 g (1³/₄ oz) wholemeal (whole-wheat) oat flour, sifted
- 15 g (¹/₂ oz) organic baking powder
- 1 teaspoon organic bourbon vanilla powder
- 100 ml (3¹/₂ fl oz) rice milk
- 50 ml (1³/₄ fl oz) mild extra virgin olive oil (or 75 ml/2¹/₄ fl oz cold-pressed organic sunflower oil)
- 4–5 tablespoons raw honey
- 2 bananas
- juice and zest of 1 lemon
- 1 tablespoon coarsely chopped walnuts

**METHOD**

Preheat the oven to 180°C (350°F/Gas 4). Lightly grease and line a loaf (bar) tin with baking paper.

Combine the flours, baking powder and vanilla in a large bowl.

In a separate bowl, beat the rice milk, olive oil and honey using an electric mixer.

Mash the bananas with a fork and add to the liquid mixture with the lemon juice and zest. Add the liquid ingredients to the flour mixture and mix well.

Pour the batter into the tin and sprinkle the surface of the cake with walnuts. Bake for 35-40 minutes, or until golden brown. Cool in the tin for 5 minutes before lifting out carefully onto a wire rack to cool completely.

*Fruit for breakfast is one of those good habits. With a few ingredients and the right combinations, you can create delicious dishes that satisfy even the most reluctant.*

*The key ingredient in this recipe is the date nectar—an excellent sugar alternative, rich in nutrients. Dates are rich in fibre, protein and minerals such as potassium, magnesium, phosphorus, selenium, calcium, sodium. They are also rich in vitamin A, B1, B2, B3, B5, B6, K and J. Its sugars are dextrose, fructose, maltose and sucrose. Date nectar has a very delicate and not intrusive flavour which gives recipes a special twist.*

*In this recipe, if desired, you can replace date nectar with honey or a spoonful of coconut sugar.*

# BANANAS WITH CARAMELIZED PEARS

(BANANE CON PERE CARAMELLATE)

GF-V

*Serves 4*

## INGREDIENTS

· 4 bananas
· juice of 1 lemon
· 2 tablespoons whole date nectar/syrup
· 3 pears (not too ripe)

· 2 tablespoons water
· 1 tablespoon Marsala dessert wine
· 1 teaspoon ground cinnamon

## METHOD

Preheat the oven to 180°C (350°F/Gas 4). Lightly grease and line a baking tray with baking paper.
Peel the bananas and split in half lengthwise. Sprinkle with the lemon juice to prevent blackening.
Place the bananas on the tray. Drizzle with 1 tablespoon of date nectar and bake for 10–15 minutes.
Meanwhile, peel and cut the pears into cubes and cook in a saucepan with 2 tablespoons of water, the
    remaining date nectar and the Marsala, until the pears are soft.
Serve the bananas warm with the pears and a sprinkling of cinnamon.

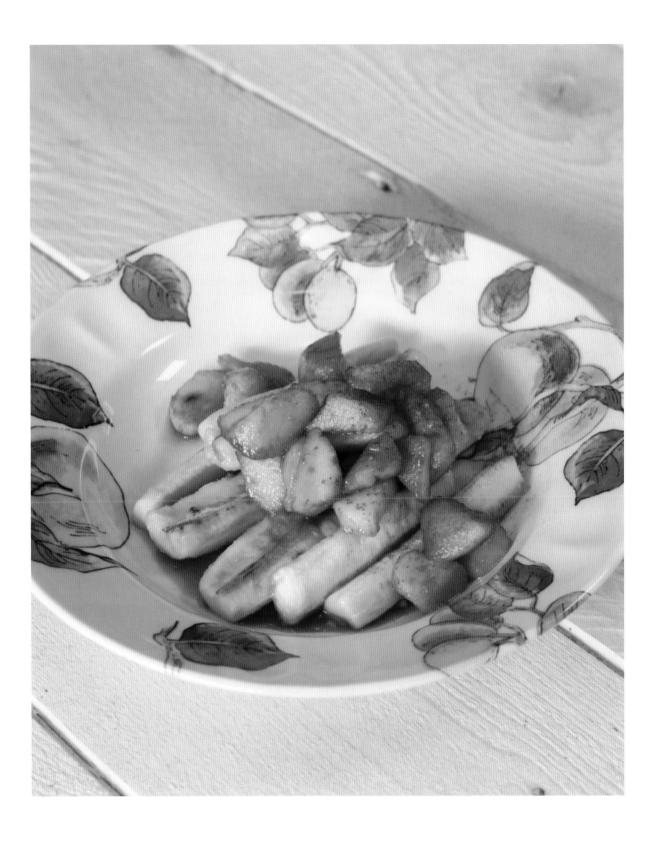

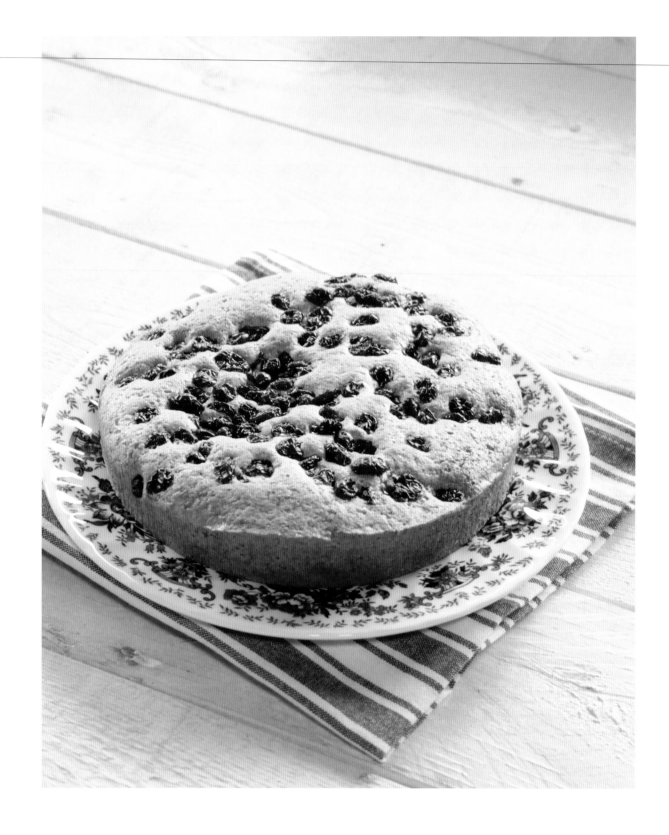

*Zucchini (courgettes), in season, and dried cranberries are the winning combination in this delicious cake—perfect for spring and summer breakfast.*

*Involving children in preparing cakes like this is a great idea because it teaches them to vary the ingredients, allows them to try different flavours and encourages them to eat more fruit and vegetables.*

# CAKE WITH ZUCCHINI AND DRIED CRANBERRIES

## (TORTA DI ZUCCHINE E MIRTILLI ROSSI ESSICCATI)

### GF-DF-VEG

### *Serves 6*

## INGREDIENTS

- 2 eggs
- 75 ml (2$^{1}/_{4}$ fl oz) mild extra virgin olive oil (or 100 ml/3$^{1}/_{2}$ fl oz cold-pressed
- organic sunflower oil)
- 80 g (2$^{3}/_{4}$ oz) raw coconut sugar
- 200 g (7 oz) brown rice flour, sifted
- 50 g (1$^{3}/_{4}$ oz) buckwheat flour, sifted
- 15 g ($^{1}/_{2}$ oz) organic baking powder
- 1 tablespoon bourbon vanilla powder
- 1 banana
- 2 zucchini (courgettes), grated
- 1 handful dried cranberries (sugar and palm oil free)

## METHOD

Preheat the oven to 180°C (350°F/Gas 4). Lightly grease and line a 22 cm (8$^{1}/_{2}$ inch) springform tin with baking paper.

Using an electric mixer, beat the eggs with the olive oil and sugar. Add the flour, baking powder and cinnamon and mix until well combined.

Peel the banana and mash in a bowl using a fork. Add the flour to the banana, along with grated zucchini. Add the dried cranberries.

Pour the batter into the tin and bake for 40 minutes, or until golden brown. Cool in the tin for 5 minutes before lifting out carefully onto a wire rack to cool completely.

*Crispy and rich in energy, these cookies are a real concentration of benefits. I make them often and share with family and friends. They are great for breakfast, dipped in milk, but also perfect for a snack to take with you to school or the office. They can keep for several days.*

*You can replace (or alternate) dried fruit according to your tastes.*

# COCOA CARROT COOKIES WITH PISTACHIOS

(BISCOTTI AL CACAO CON CAROTE E PISTACCHI)

V

## Serves 6

### INGREDIENTS

- 100 g (7 oz) wholemeal (whole-wheat) flour, sifted (or brown rice flour, for a gluten-free recipe)
- 150 g (5$^1$/$_2$ oz) pistachio flour
- 100 g (3$^1$/$_2$ oz) cornflakes
- 1 tablespoon raw cocoa powder
- 3 tablespoons raw coconut sugar
- 1 teaspoon organic baking powder
- pinch of sea salt
- 2 grated carrots
- 50 ml (1$^3$/$_4$ fl oz) extra virgin olive oil or 100 ml (3$^1$/$_2$ fl oz) cold-pressed sunflower oil
- rice milk, to taste
- 1 handful chopped pistachios or other dried fruit, to your taste

### METHOD

Preheat the oven to 180°C (350°F/ Gas 4). Line a baking tray with baking paper.

Combine the flours, cornflakes, cocoa powder, coconut sugar, baking powder, salt, grated carrots in a bowl.

Add the oil and mix the ingredients using an electric mixer. Add just enough milk to make a soft dough.

With moistened hands, form small balls. Flatten and place on the baking tray.

Place the pistachios or other chopped dried fruit on each cookie and bake for 20 minutes, or until lightly golden. Remove from the oven and leave to cool on a wire rack.

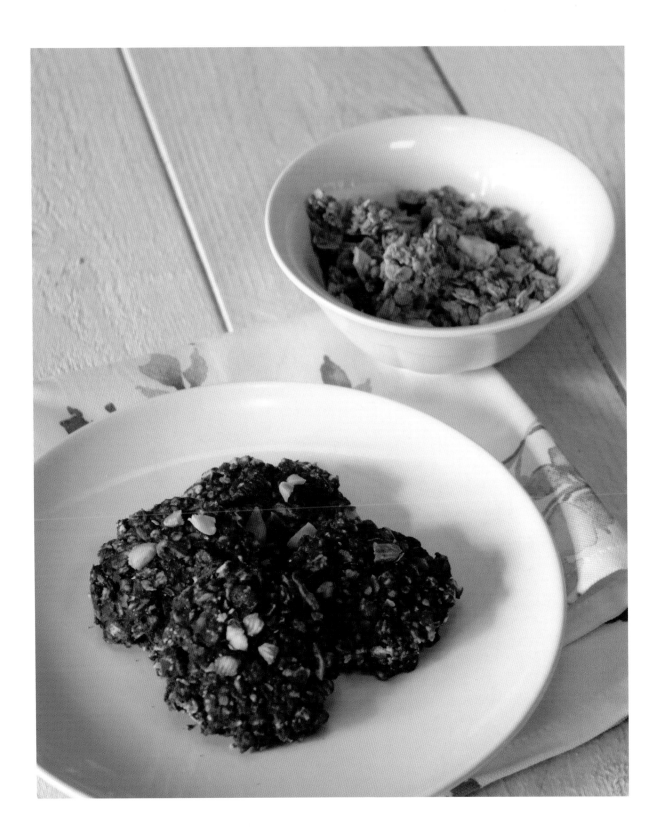

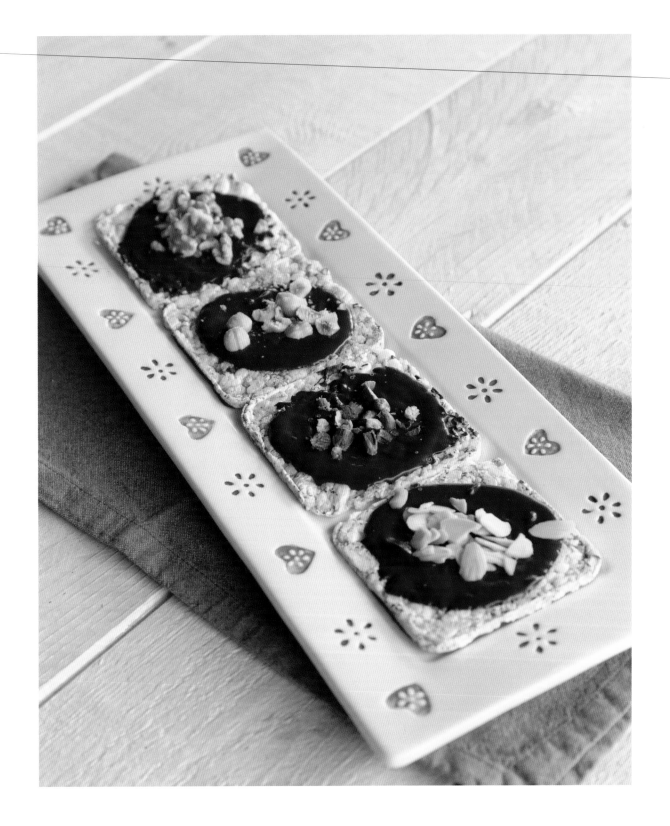

*The multigrain cakes (brown, corn, buckwheat, farro or kamut) are a very light and healthy idea and perfect for spreading with honey, jam and other delicacies.*

# CEREAL CAKES WITH CHOCOLATE GLAZE

(GALLETTE AI CEREALI CON GLASSA DI CIOCCOLATO)

V

*Makes 15*

**INGREDIENTS**

· 200 g (7 oz) 70% dark chocolate
· 15 rice cakes or corn thins

· 50 g (1³/₄ oz) coarsely chopped toasted hazelnuts (or almonds)

**METHOD**

Melt the chocolate in a double boiler. Leave to cool for 3–5 minutes.

Pour 1 or 2 tablespoons of melted chocolate over each cake (the amount depends on the size of the cereal cakes).

Sprinkle with the chopped hazelnuts. Leave to cool completely, then serve.

*A soft, moist cake with a delicate flavour. Ideal for dipping in milk, it is perfect also as a dessert after a light meal. In this recipe, pistachio is the ingredient that makes the difference.*

# FROSTED CARROT CAKE

(TORTA GLASSATA DI CAROTE)

GF-VEG

*Serves 6-8*

## INGREDIENTS

- 100 g (3$^1$/$_2$ oz) pistachios
- 50 g (1$^3$/$_4$ oz) toasted whole almonds
- 80 g (2$^3$/$_4$ oz) dark brown sugar
- 3 carrots
- pinch of sea salt
- 1 egg

- 150 g (5$^1$/$_2$ oz) brown rice flour, sifted
- 15 g ($^1$/$_2$ oz) organic baking powder
- 100 g (3$^1$/$_2$ oz) 80% dark chocolate
- 1 orange zest
- 2 tablespoons sliced almonds

## METHOD

Preheat the oven to 180°C (350°F/Gas 4). Lightly grease and line a 22 cm (8$^1$/$_2$ inch) springform tin with baking paper.

In a blender, process the pistachios and almonds with the sugar and set aside.

Peel and grate the carrots and mix with a pinch of salt. Add the egg, flour and baking powder and mix quickly. Add to the pistachio and almond mixture.

Pour the batter into the baking tin. Bake for 40 minutes, or until lightly golden.

Meanwhile, melt the chocolate in a double boiler and add the orange zest.

When the cake is still warm, pour the chocolate glaze over and sprinkle with the sliced almonds.

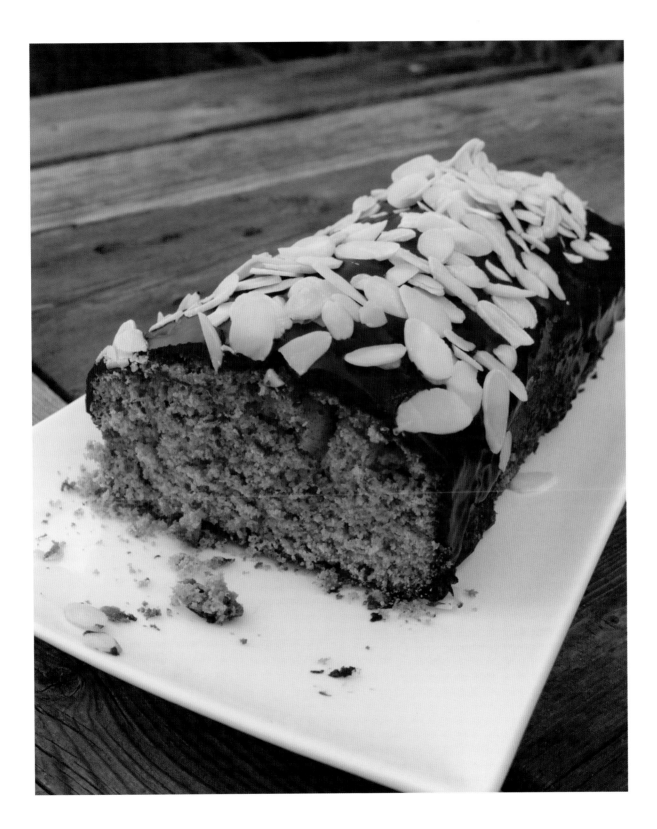

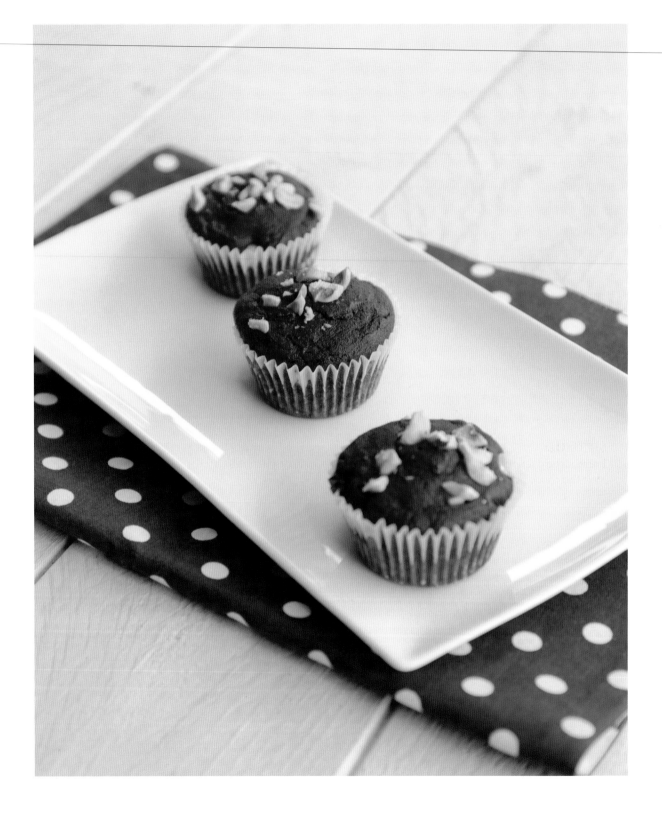

*Naturally dairy-free, these small cakes can also be gluten-free if you use brown rice flour. I have used raw dark 90% chocolate because I think bitter chocolate gives a very special taste to cakes. If 90% raw chocolate is not your thing you can use raw 70% dark chocolate. These are very easy and quick to make.*

# HAZELNUT SMALL CAKES

(TORTINE DI NOCCIOLE)

DF-VEG

*Makes 8–10*

## INGREDIENTS

· 100 g (3¹/₂ oz) 90% raw dark chocolate
· 4 tablespoons organic date nectar/syrup (or 2–3 tablespoons raw honey)
· 1 tablespoon raw cocoa powder
· 150 g (5¹/₂ oz) chopped toasted hazelnuts
· 150 g (5¹/₂ oz) wholemeal (whole-wheat) flour, sifted

· 15 g (¹/₂ oz) organic baking powder
· 140 ml 4³/₄ fl oz) water
· 50 ml (1³/₄ fl oz) mild extra virgin olive oil (or 75 ml/2¹/₄ fl oz organic cold-pressed sunflower oil)
· 1 egg
· pinch of sea salt

## METHOD

Preheat the oven to 180°C (350°F/Gas 4). Lightly grease ten muffin holes.

Melt the chocolate in a double boiler.

Using an electric mixer, mix the date nectar, cocoa, 100 g (3¹/₂ oz) chopped hazelnuts, flour and baking powder.

Add the rice milk, oil, egg, pinch of salt and mix for about 2 minutes.

Pour the mixture into the muffin holes and sprinkle with 50 g (1³/₄ oz) coarsely chopped hazelnuts.

Bake for 15 minutes, or until the muffins are risen and lightly golden. Leave in the pan for a few minutes, then transfer to a wire rack to cool.

*These honey cakes are just divine. Full of flavour and very nourishing, they are perfect in winter when I prepare them with homemade marmalade, made with Sicilian red oranges. Spices enhance the flavour of jam and add an aroma that is the hallmark of these stunning small cakes.*

# HONEY CAKES WITH MARMALADE

(TORTINE AL MIELE CON MARMELLATA)

DF-GF-VEG

*Makes 8–10*

## INGREDIENTS

- 150 ml (5 fl oz) water
- 100 g (3½ oz) raw honey
- 50 g (1¾ oz) raw brown sugar
- 100 g (3½ oz) raw brown sugar
- 1 teaspoon ground cinnamon
- 1 teaspoon ground nutmeg

- 1 beaten egg
- 300 g (10½ oz) brown rice flour, sifted
- 15 g (½ oz) organic baking powder
- 3 tablespoons mild extra virgin olive oil (or organic cold-pressed sunflower oil)
- 150 g (5½ oz) marmalade

## METHOD

Preheat the oven to 180°C (350°F/Gas 4). Lightly grease ten muffin holes.

Heat the water, honey and sugar in a saucepan over medium heat. Bring to the boil and cook until you get a syrup. Remove from the heat, add the spices and allow to cool.

Pour the syrup into a bowl. Add the beaten egg, flour, baking powder, oil and stir to combine.

Pour the batter into a muffin mold and leave to cool. Spoon a tablespoon of marmalade or sugar-free jam over each muffin hole.

Bake for 15 minutes, or until lightly golden. Leave in the pan for a few minutes, then transfer to a wire rack to cool.

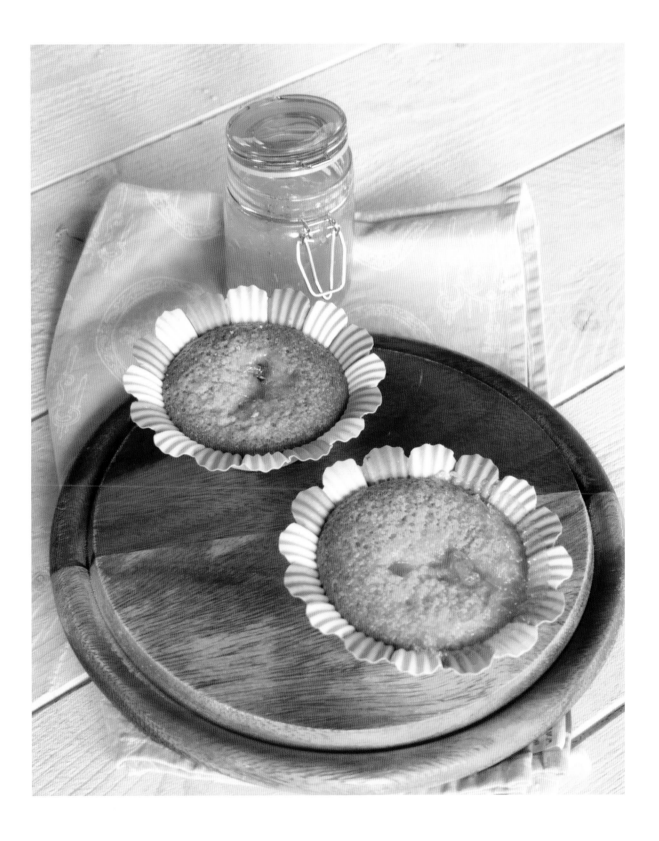

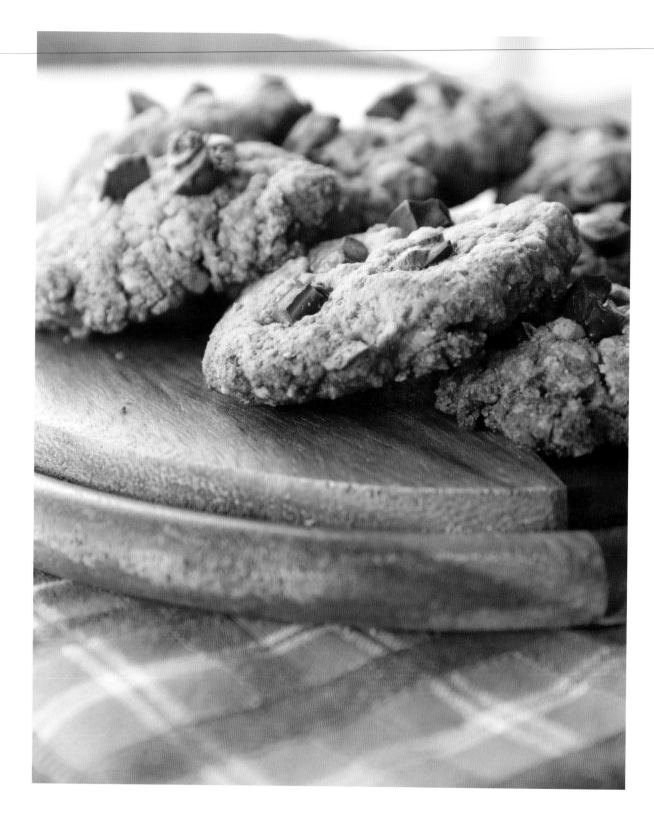

*This recipe will amaze you. The secret to the success is the excellent quality of flour and, especially, of cereal flakes (also preferably wholegrain). Of course, you can replace chopped chocolate with nuts. The amount of oil and water also depends on the type of flour used (if the flour is not rough, the quantity decreases). Because these cookies are very quick and easy to prepare, I suggest you make small quantities to be enjoyed within two days, so that their freshness and crispness remain intact.*

# OAT COOKIES WITH DARK CHOCOLATE FLAKES

## (BISCOTTONI DI AVENA CON SCAGLIE DI CIOCCOLATO FONDENTE)

EF-DF-VEG

*Makes about 10–12 (it depends on the size you size you make the cookies)*

## INGREDIENTS

- 200 g (7 oz) wholemeal (whole-wheat) oat flour
- 50 g (1¾ oz) wholemeal (whole-wheat) farro (or kamut) flour
- 150 g (5½ oz) barley or oats flakes, sugar-free
- 1 tablespoon organic baking powder
- 4 tablespoons date nectar/syrup
- pinch of sea salt
- 100 ml (3½ fl oz) cold-pressed sunflower oil
- 50 ml (1¾ fl oz) water (optional)
- 50 g (1¾ oz) chopped dark chocolate

## METHOD

Preheat the oven to 180°C (350°F/Gas 4). Line a baking tray with baking paper.

Combine the flours, barley or oats flakes, baking powder, date nectar and pinch of salt in a bowl. Add the oil and mix to combine. Add extra water if the dough is dry.

With moistened hands, picked up a little dough, form into balls and place on the baking tray.

Flatten the balls, and sprinkle some of the chopped chocolate on top. Bake for 15 minutes, or until lightly golden. Stand on tray for 5 minutes to cool before transferring to a wire rack to cool completely.

*When Dad came home with the first boxes of juicy oranges of the season, my sisters and I were all happy. We already knew that Mom would make so much orange marmalade and that, part of this, would be used for filling luscious tarts and other sweets.*

*'Oranges for breakfast!' my mother would call out, getting us get out of bed without much effort. Waiting for us in the kitchen, there was always something baked with the scent of oranges, tarts, cakes or cookies.*

*Among the many sweet awakenings of my winter childhood, I will keep this memory. Those moments have inspired this cake made with all natural ingredients that has, as key ingredient, the fruit symbol of Sicily to which my mother was able to give a fitting tribute.*

# ORANGE CAKE

(TORTA DI ARANCE)

DF-GF-VEG

*Serves 6-8*

## INGREDIENTS

- 200 g (7 oz) brown rice flour, sifted
- 50 g (1³/₄ oz) almond flour, sifted
- 15 g (¹/₂ oz) organic baking powder
- 2 oranges, plus juice and zest
- 4–5 tablespoons raw honey
- pinch of sea salt
- 2 beaten eggs
- 50 ml (1³/₄ fl oz) mild extra virgin olive oil (or 4 tablespoons organic cold-pressed sunflower oil)
- 4 tablespoons rice milk

## METHOD

Preheat the oven to 180°C (350°F/Gas 4). Lightly grease and line a 22 cm (8¹/₂ inch) springform tin with baking paper.

Combine the sifted flours, baking powder, orange juice and zest, honey and a pinch of salt in a large bowl. Add 2 beaten eggs, the olive oil and milk and mix the ingredients until creamy and smooth.

Pour the batter into the tin.

Slice the oranges. Put the oranges over the dough and bake for 35–40 minutes, or until a skewer inserted into the centre comes out clean. Leave to cool in the tin for about 5 minutes before turning out onto a wire rack to cool completely.

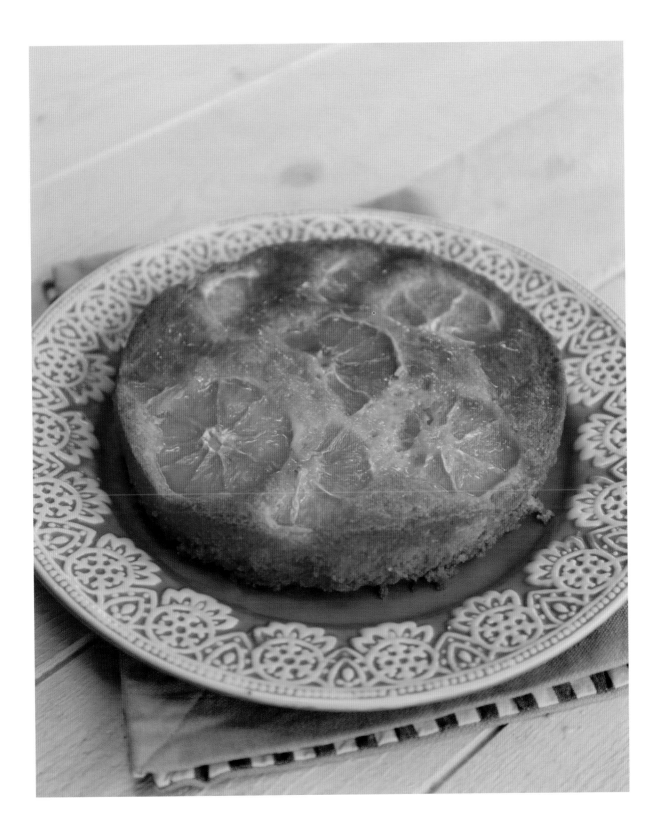

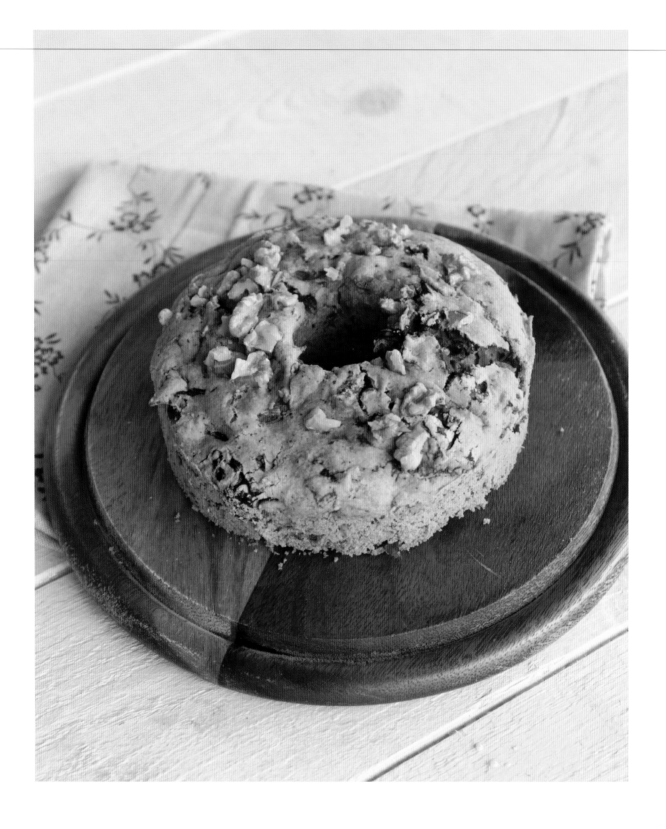

*The versatility of radicchio makes it one of my favourite vegetables, and it's perfect for sweet cakes.*
*The bitterness of the radicchio is tempered by the gentle sweetness of dark chocolate and carrots. The latter,*
*together with toasted hazelnuts, keeps this rustic cake moist and makes it ideal to be served as an afternoon snack.*

# RADICCHIO AND CHOCOLATE CAKE

(TORTA DI RADICCHIO E CIOCCOLATO)

GF-DF-VEG

*Serves 6-8*

## INGREDIENTS

- 50 g (1³/₄ oz) 70% dark chocolate, chopped
- 50 g (2 oz) 60% dark chocolate, chopped
- 1 egg
- 4 tablespoons mild extra virgin olive oil (or 100 ml/3¹/₂ fl oz organic cold-pressed sunflower oil)
- 80 g (2³/₄ oz) raw coconut sugar
- 250 g (9 oz) brown rice flour, sifted
- 15 g (¹/₂ oz) organic baking powder
- 100 g (3¹/₂ oz) toasted hazelnut flour
- 100 g (3¹/₂ oz) grated carrots
- 150 g (5¹/₂ oz) chopped round radicchio
- 100 g (3¹/₂ oz) chopped walnuts

## METHOD

Preheat the oven to 180°C (350°F/Gas 4). Lightly grease and line a 16 cm (6¹/₄ inch) round cake tin with baking paper.

Beat the egg white until stiff. In a separate bowl, beat the yolk with the oil and sugar until the mixture is foamy.

Add the chocolate?, rice flour, baking powder, hazelnut flour (just blend hazelnuts in a food processor), grated carrots, chopped radicchio and stir. Stir in the egg white, mixing from the bottom upwards.

Pour the dough into the tin and bake for 40 minutes, or until lightly golden. While still warm, decorate with a sprinkling of chopped walnuts.

*This cake, with a very special aroma, is one of my favourite winter breakfasts. Adding aromatic plants to sweet recipes is a good tip I learnt from my mother.*

*This cake, also ideal for a classic afternoon tea, remains very soft and is perfect for a burst of energy in the early morning.*

# ROSEMARY AND ALMOND CAKE

(TORTA DI MANDORLE E ROSMARINO)

VEG

### Serves 6-8

## INGREDIENTS

- 75 ml (2¹/₄ fl oz) mild extra virgin olive oil (or 100 ml/3¹/₂ fl oz organic cold-pressed sunflower oil)
- 1 rosemary sprig
- 150 g (5¹/₂ oz) wholemeal (whole-wheat) flour, sifted
- 80 g (2³/₄ oz) almond flour
- 80 g (2³/₄ oz) cornstarch (cornmeal)
- 15 g (¹/₂ oz) organic baking powder
- 50 g (1³/₄ oz) raw brown sugar

- 1 beaten egg
- juice and zest of 1 red orange
- 100 g (3¹/₂ oz) 80% chopped dark chocolate or Modica Aztec chocolate
- 100 ml (3 fl oz) apple juice, no sugars added
- 150 ml (5 fl oz) rice milk
- 1 handful pistachios, sliced almonds or other dried fruit

## METHOD

Preheat the oven to 180°C (350°F/Gas 4). Lightly grease and line a 22 cm (8¹/₂ inch) springform tin with baking paper.

Heat the oil and rosemary needles in a saucepan over medium heat for 3 minutes. Remove from the heat and leave to cool.

Combine the wholemeal flour, almond flour, cornstarch and brown sugar. Add the beaten egg, juice and orange zest and chocolate flakes.

Strain the oil using a sieve to remove the rosemary. Add the apple juice and rice milk.

Add the liquid ingredients to solid. Pour the batter into the baking tin. Cover with 1 handful dried fruit of your choice.

Bake for 40 minutes, or until lightly golden and a skewer inserted into the centre comes out clean. Leave to cool in the tin for 5 minutes before turning out onto a wire rack to cool completely.

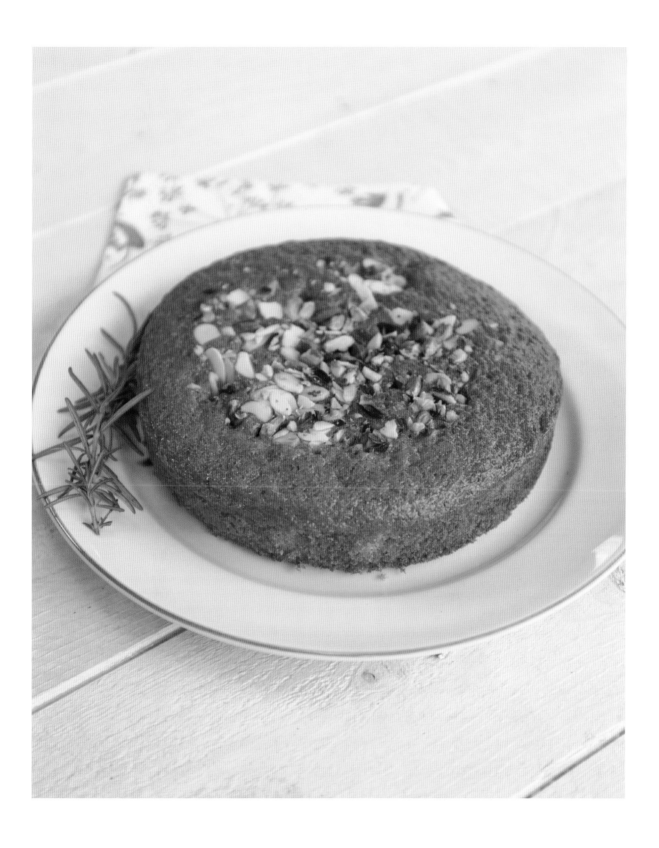

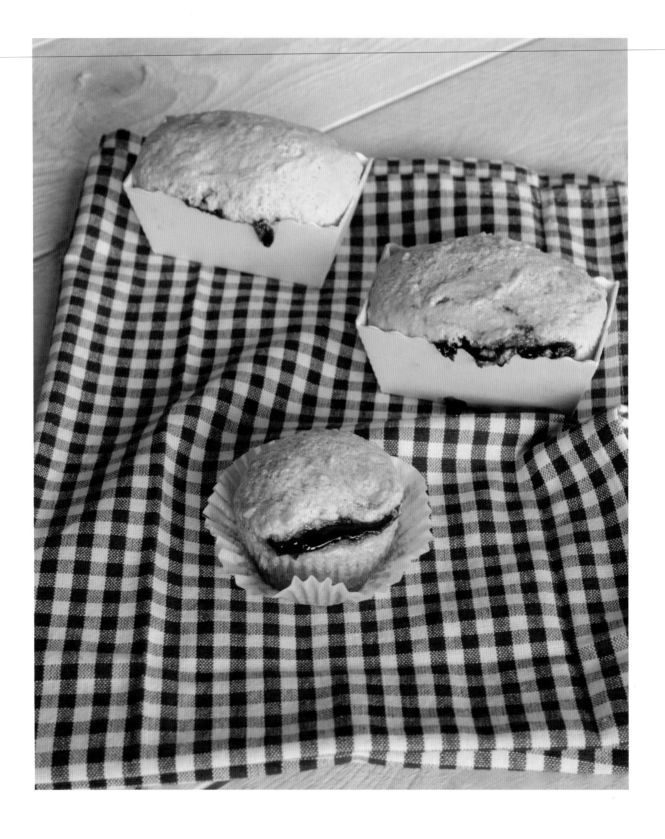

*These cakes have an exquisite taste and texture. When accompanied by ice cream or hot chocolate, they are also ideal for a sweet afternoon break.*

*The fresh blackberries, when baked in the oven, become a creamy jam that makes the inside of the cakes moist and delicious. Perfect to be served in individual portions, they can be prepared in both the muffin or mini-loaf molds.*

# SMALL CAKES WITH BLACKBERRIES

(TORTINE ALLE MORE)

VEG

*Makes 6-8*

## INGREDIENTS

- 200 g (7 oz) wholemeal (whole-wheat) kamut or farro flour, sifted
- 100 g (3$\frac{1}{2}$ oz) cashew flour
- 2 teaspoon organic baking powder
- 4 tablespoons whole date nectar juice
- pinch of sea salt
- 1 teaspoon ground cinnamon
- 100 ml (3$\frac{1}{2}$ fl oz) rice or soy yoghurt, sugar-free
- 50 ml (1$\frac{3}{4}$ fl oz) mild extra virgin olive oil (or 100 ml/3 fl oz cold-pressed sunflower oil)
- 100 ml (3$\frac{1}{2}$ fl oz) warm water
- 100 g (3$\frac{1}{2}$ oz) fresh blackberries
- juice of 1 lemon

## METHOD

Preheat the oven to 180°C (350°F/Gas 4). Lightly grease eight muffin holes.

Combine the flour sifted with the baking powder, the date nectar, salt, cinnamon and yoghurt in a bowl. Add the olive oil and water, stirring constantly until the mixture is smooth.

Mash the blackberries with the tines of a fork and drizzle with the lemon juice.

Add 1 teaspoon mashed blackberries into each muffin hole. Divide the batter between six to eight muffin holes.

Bake for 30 minutes, or until lightly golden and a skewer inserted into the centre comes out clean. Leave to cool in the tin for 5 minutes before turning out onto a wire rack to cool completely.

*A classic breakfast cake, enriched with simple but healthy and nutritious ingredients. The raw honey makes the cake very soft and delicately scented. The puffed rice is crispy and children love it.*

# WHOLE LOAF CAKE WITH YOGHURT

(TORTA INTEGRALE ALLO YOGURT)

DF-VEG

*Serves 6–8*

## INGREDIENTS

- 2 large eggs
- 3 tablespoons mild extra virgin olive oil (or 100 ml/3 fl oz cold-pressed
- sunflower oil)
- 100 g (3½ oz) rice or soy yoghurt
- zest of 1 lemon

- 4 tablespoons raw honey
- 250 g (9 oz) wholemeal (wholewheat) flour (or wholemeal Farro, Kamut flour), sifted
- 15 g (½ oz) organic baking powder
- 100 g (3½ oz) puffed brown rice

## METHOD

Preheat the oven to 180°C (350°F/Gas 4). Lightly grease and line a loaf (bar) tin with baking paper.

Using a blender or food processor, add all of the ingredients except for the puffed rice and process for 2 minutes.

Pour the batter into the prepared tin. Cover with the puffed brown rice and bake for 35 minutes. Leave to cool in the tin for 5 minutes before turning out onto a wire rack to cool completely.

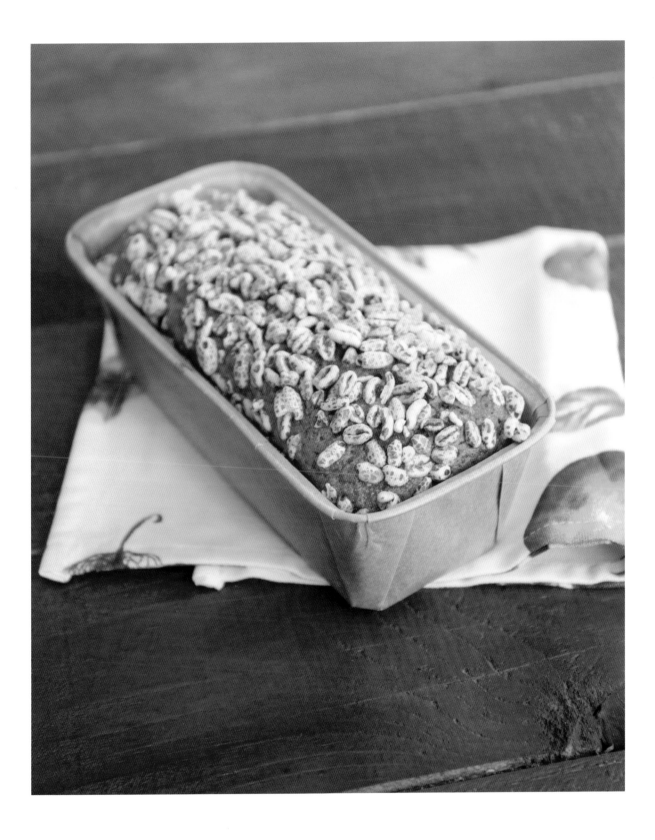

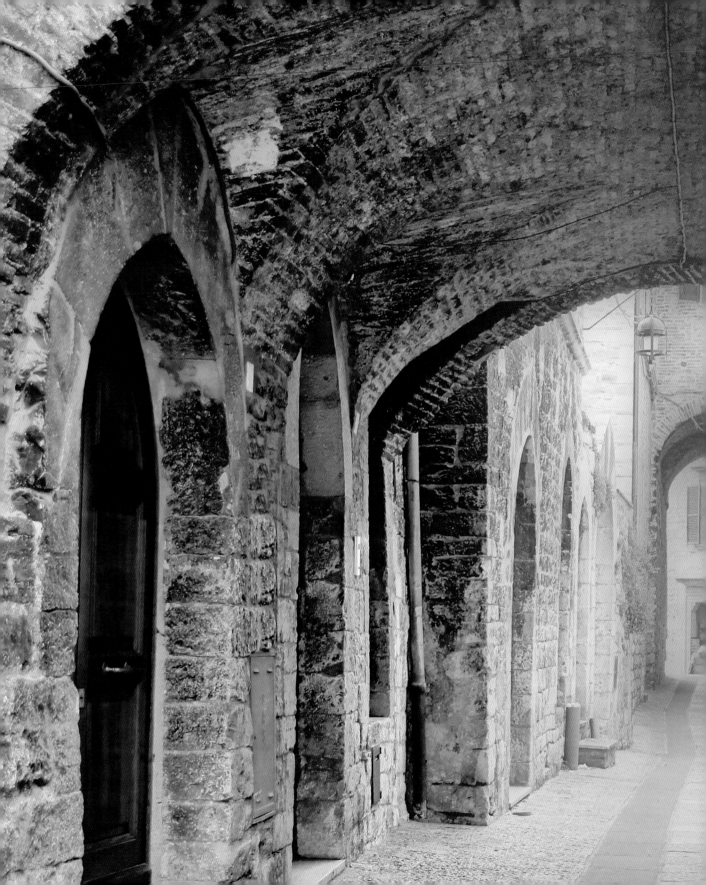

# APPETIZERS & BRUNCH

The so-called Italian "antipasto" (appetizer-starter. Literally: "Before the meal") dates back to the tables of ancient Rome. The Romans, lovers of good food, introduced something delicious and appetizing before starting the meal. Lovers of a mostly vegetarian diet, they were aware of the importance of starting a meal with vegetables and salads to prepare the stomach to receive the other courses (the tables of the rich meals were very elaborate and lengthy).

After the fall of the Roman Empire (and throughout the Middle Ages) the starter fell into disuse and reappeared on Italian tables in the Italian Renaissance.

The appetizers in this book are a healthy and tasty option not only for main meals but also for an informal brunch or for a snack.

Bread is one of the key ingredients of Italian antipasti. Bruschetta and crostoni are an ideal base for tasty recipes. I always choose rustic bread with wholemeal (whole-wheat) flour quality. This type of bread is kept perfectly for several days and if heated in the oven, brings out more of its quality.

Vegetables and salads are another great option as a starter or informal brunch.

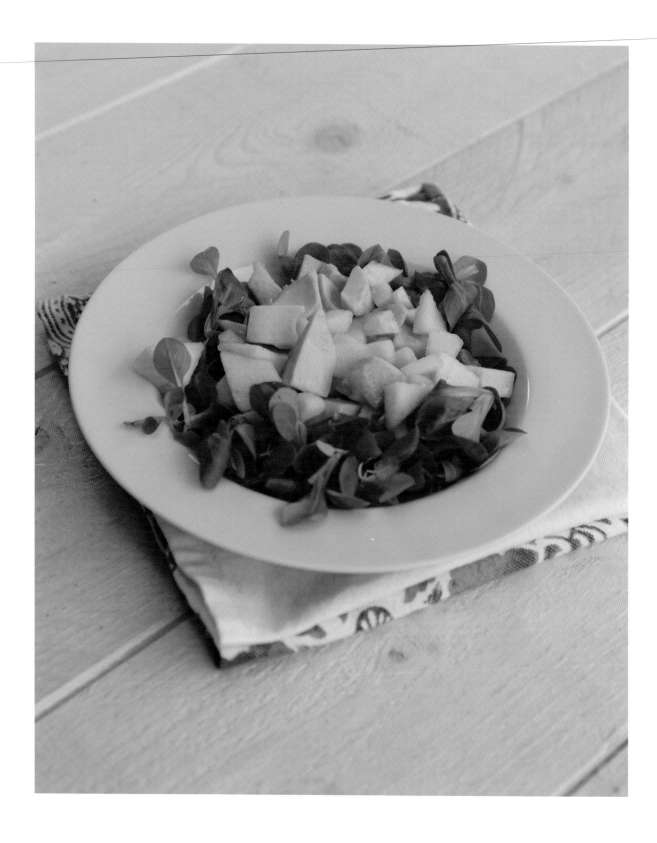

Rich in minerals and vitamins (not to be confused with the Valeriana officinalis), Valerian is one of the key ingredients of this salad. Of course, when it is not in season, you can replace with other vegetables, although its taste matches perfectly with avocado.

Since I discovered that one of the major growers and exporters of avocado in Europe is Sicilian, and that his company is not far from my house, I admit to consuming avocadoes with a lot more enthusiasm.

Rich in unsaturated fats and omega-3, avocado stimulates the production of good cholesterol (HDL) and improve bad levels of cholesterol (LDL).

Avocado is also rich in Vitamin A and E, powerful antioxidants which help against aging skin. Its Vitamin D content helps the body absorb calcium and phosphorus.

# AVOCADO SALAD

(INSALATA DI AVOCADO)

V

*Serves 2*

## INGREDIENTS

- 3 tablespoons extra virgin olive oil
- juice and zest of 1 lemon
- pinch of sea salt
- white pepper, to taste
- 1 ripe avocado
- 2 green apples
- 2 handful valerian leaves (or other seasonal salad)

## METHOD

In a salad bowl, emulsify the olive oil with the juice of lemon and pinch of salt. Once you have obtained an opaque and more dense emulsion, add the grated lemon zest.

Cut the avocado into 4 wedges and remove the peel. Cut into cubes and soak it in the citronette.

Peel and cut the apples and mix well with avocado. Add the valerian.

Mix well and refrigerate for about 10 minutes before serving.

*I only discovered vegan cheese a few years ago. I am not intolerant to lactose and I love Italian cheeses but I also adore the lightness of vegan alternatives. They are also perfect for people who want to discover more delicate flavours and new textures.*

*This delicious vegan bruschetta is easy to make and alternate with seasonal vegetables.*

# BRUSCHETTA WITH RED ONION, ARTICHOKES AND VEGAN CHEESE

(BRUSCHETTA CON CIPOLLA ROSSA, CARCIOFI E FORMAGGIO VEGANO)

V

*Serves 4*

### INGREDIENTS

· 200 g (7 oz) artichokes hearts
· 250 g (9 oz) vegan cheese (I generally buy rice cheese), diced
· 1 red onion, roughly chopped
· extra virgin olive oil, to taste
· pinch of sea salt
· 4 slices of country-style bread

### METHOD

Wash the artichokes hearts. Place in a saucepan of salted water over medium heat and boil for about 15 minutes. Drain and return to the pan with some olive oil for 5 minutes. Allow to cool, then cut into pieces.

Preheat oven to 180°C (350°F/Gas 4). Line a baking tray with baking paper.

Combine the cheese, red onion, artichokes and olive oil in a bowl.

Arrange the bread slices on the baking tray and bake for 5–8 minutes, or until the cheese begins to melt.

Remove from the oven and top the bread slices with the artichoke salad and serve immediately.

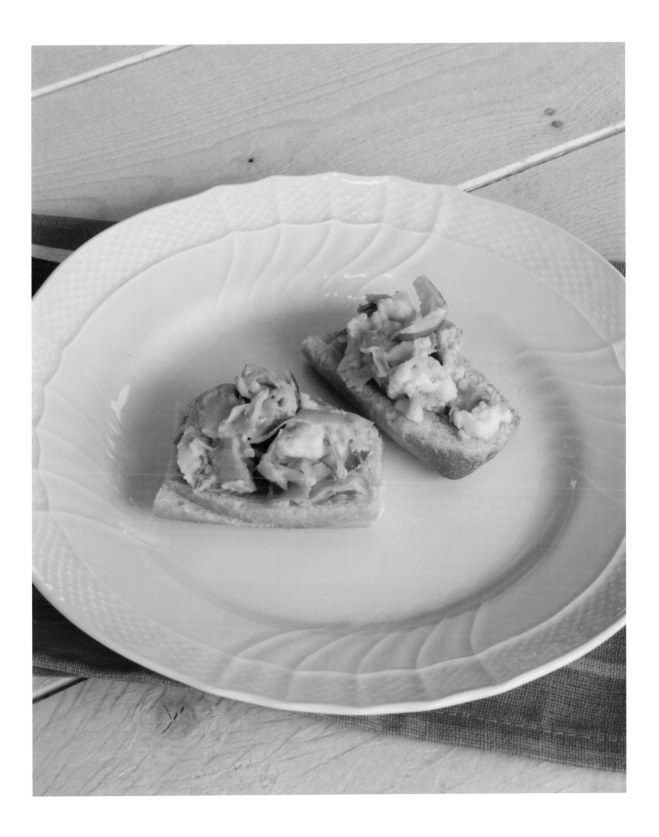

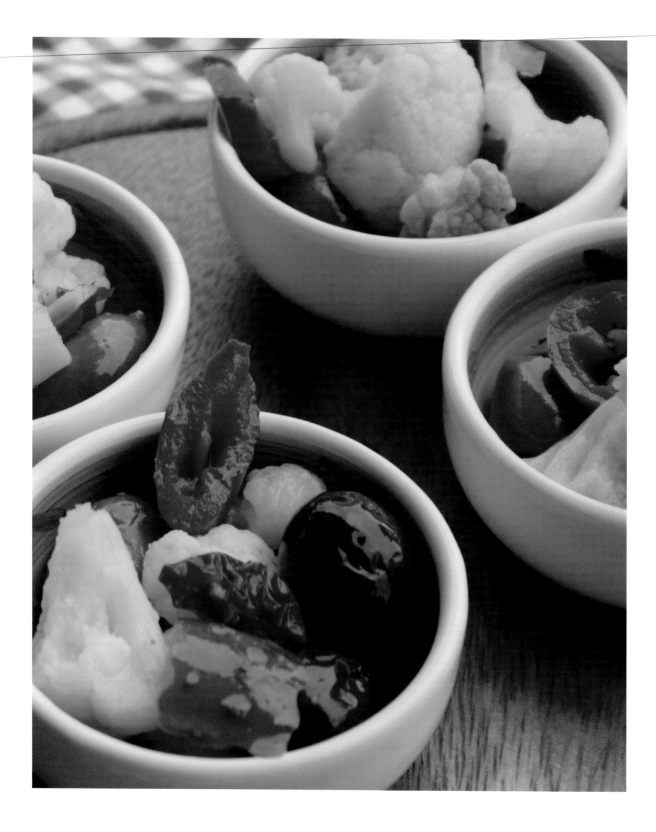

*As a child, I did not like cauliflower. I didn't like the taste, and I assumed that therefore, it could not be nutritional. The prejudices we have about certain foods can sometimes mean we neglect them in favour of other more attractive ingredients.*

*This cauliflower salad is simple but rich in flavous, and is best consumed in autumn and winter. A quality oil, excellent black olives and, of course, a fresh cauliflower, make this recipe special.*

*Usually, when cooking cauliflower, it is recommended you add a tablespoon of white or apple cider vinegar to avoid the unpleasant smell, but if the vegetable is organic you'll hardly notice the smell.*

# CAULIFLOWER SALAD WITH OLIVES

(INSALATA DI CAVOLFIORE CON OLIVE)

V

### *Serves 2*

## INGREDIENTS

· 1 small cauliflower
· 1 parsley sprig
· 10 black olives, pitted, halved
· 1 garlic clove, crushed
· extra virgin olive oil, to taste
· sea salt, to taste

## METHOD

Place the cauliflower on a cutting board. With a knife, remove the stem and the outer leaves. Divide the cauliflower into florets (if they are large, cut them in half).

Place the florets in a colander and rinse them with cold water one by one. Steam the florets for 30 minutes (or boil them in salted water for 15 minutes).

Remove the parsley stalks and chop the leaves.

Place the parsley and olives in a bowl. Add the crushed garlic, oil, pepper, salt and let sit for about 10 minutes.

Remove the garlic from the parsley and pour the mixture over the cauliflower. Stir gently and serve.

*Enriching your diet with ancient cereals (they are at the core of the Mediterranean diet) is not only a healthy habit but a pleasure. Farro is one of the oldest cereals, a hero of the Italian tables and, now, available everywhere.*

*Wholegrains are the best choice but, often a lack of time leads many to avoid these foods because they require a long soak (about 6–8 hours).*

*Hulled farro (or barley) is, of course, the healthiest choice. When you short on time, choose a good-quality (possible, organic) pearled or semi-pearled grain. They do not need to soak. This recipe is prepared with the semi-pearled farro to meet the needs of those who do not have time, but I encourage you to try hulled farro or other unprocessed cereals.*

*Caramelized hazelnuts are the twist in this delicious salad that can be a main dish—perfect for a brunch.*

# CEREAL FRESH SALAD

(INSALATA DI CEREALI)

V

*Serves 4*

## INGREDIENTS

· 300 g (10¹/₂ oz) semi-pearled farro (or barley)
· 1 head of radicchio
· 1 fennel
· extra virgin olive oil, to taste
· sea salt and pepper, to taste
· 1 tablespoon apple cider vinegar
· 100 g (3¹/₂ oz) toasted chopped hazelnuts
· 1 tablespoon raw coconut sugar

## METHOD

Cook the farro in boiling salted water, according to the directions on the packaging.
Wash and clean the radicchio and fennel and cut them into strips.
Put the vegetables in a bowl and add the olive oil, salt, pepper and apple cider vinegar. Toss to combine.
In a frying pan over medium heat, caramelize the hazelnuts with the coconut sugar.
Drain the farro and serve with the vegetables and caramelized hazelnuts.

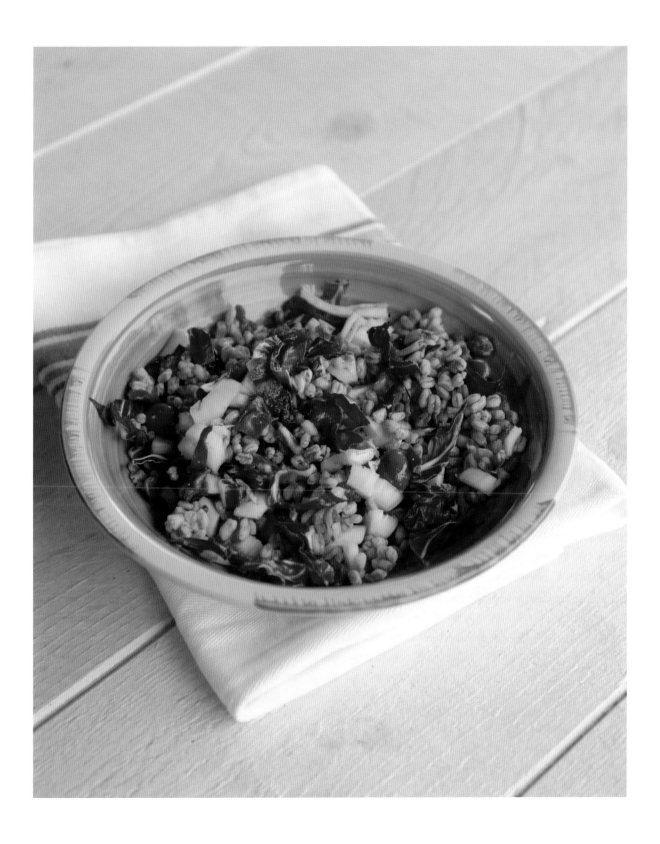

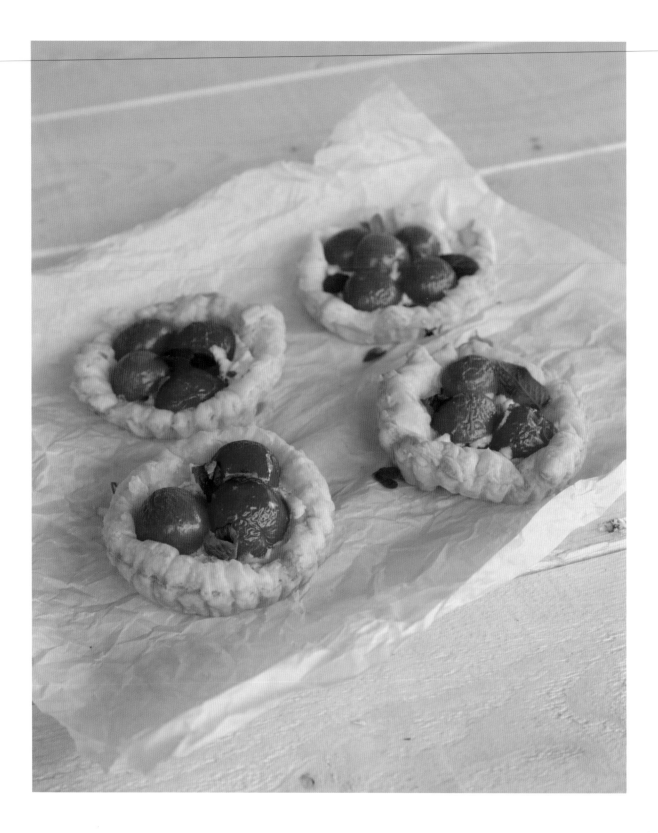

*Robiola is one of my favorite Italian cheeses. Available in the best supermarkets and Italian food shops, it has an incredible creamy texture and a delicate taste that makes it perfect for many preparations.*

*A product of Piedmont (North Italy), Robiola is made with sheep's milk. The most renowned and protected designation of origin is Roccaverano's Robiola.*

# CHERRY TOMATOES WITH SOFT CHEESE IN PUFF PASTRY

(SFOGLIA DI POMODORINI CON FORMAGGIO CREMOSO)

EF-VEG

*Serves 4*

## INGREDIENTS

- 200 g (7 oz) Robiola cheese
- 2 tablespoons Parmigiano cheese, grated
- 160 ml (5¼ fl oz) extra virgin olive oil
- sea salt and pepper, to taste
- 15 cherry tomatoes
- 1 handful oregano
- 1 handful flat-leaf (Italian) parsley
- 3 tablespoons Pecorino Romano, grated
- 50 g (1¾ oz) toasted hazelnuts (or almonds)
- 250 g (7 oz) puff pastry, palm oil free

## METHOD

Preheat the oven to 180°C (350°F/Gas 4). Grease 4 round, fluted, loose-based flan tins.

Mix the Robiola, Parmigiano, Pecorino, 1 tablespoon extra virgin olive oil, salt and pepper and set aside.

Cut the cherry tomatoes in half, spoon out the insides and filled with cream cheese.

Using a blender or food processor, blend the parsley and oregano with the hazelnuts, cheese mixture and 120 ml (4 fl oz) of oil.

Line the flan tins with the pastry, prick the surface and spread with the basil pesto. Place a cherry tomato, with the stuffed part facing downward, in each flan tin. Dress with a tablespoon of the remaining oil and garnish with basil and fresh oregano leaves, if you like.

Bake for 25–30 minutes. Allow to cool before serving.

*For Italians, bread is an essential food. The rustic bread, prepared with high-quality flour, is the ingredient that makes a difference in this recipe. Usually, I only use dried legumes. However, sometimes, when I have to prepare a quick appetizer or snack, I choose organic chickpeas or beans in jar.*

*This recipe is made special by a great Sicilian extra virgin olive oil that enhances the taste of rustic bread.*

# CHICKPEA BRUSCHETTA

### (BRUSCHETTA DI CECI)

V

*Serves 4*

## INGREDIENTS

- 300 g (10$\frac{1}{2}$ oz) chickpeas
- 1 red onion, sliced
- chopped flat-leaf (Italian) parsley, to taste
- pinch of sea salt
- juice of 1 lemon
- 2 tablespoons tahini sauce
- 2 tablespoons apple cider vinegar
- extra virgin olive oil, to taste
- 4 rustic style bread slices

## METHOD

Preheat the oven to 180°C (350°F/Gas 4). Line a baking tray with baking paper.

Combine the chickpeas, onion, parsley and a pinch of salt in a bowl.

Combine the lemon juice, tahini sauce, apple cider vinegar, and olive oil in a separate bowl. Add to the chickpea mixture and toss gently to coat.

Place the bread slices on the baking tray and bake for 5 minutes.

Arrange the bread slices on a serving dish and top each slice with 1 tablespoon of the chickpea mixture. Serve immediately.

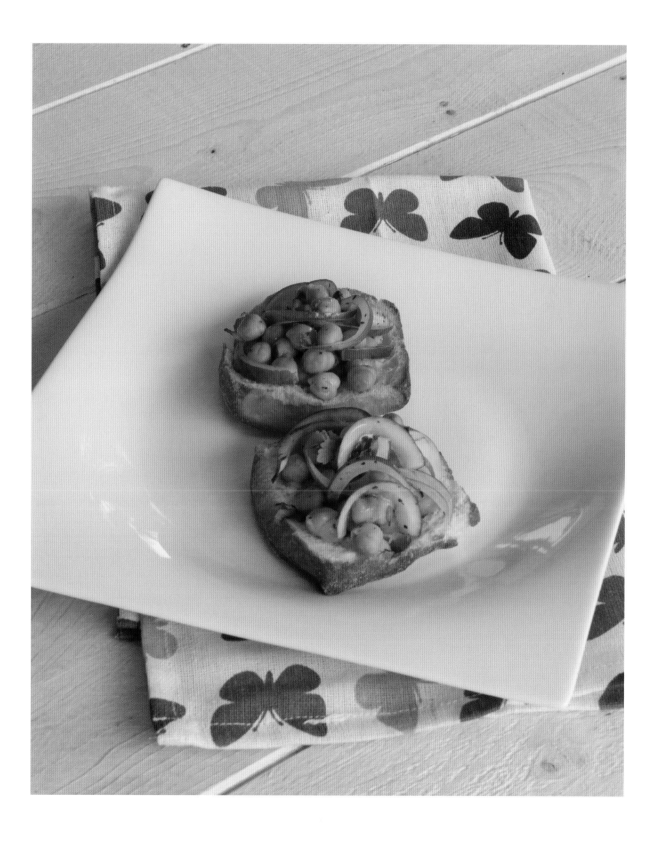

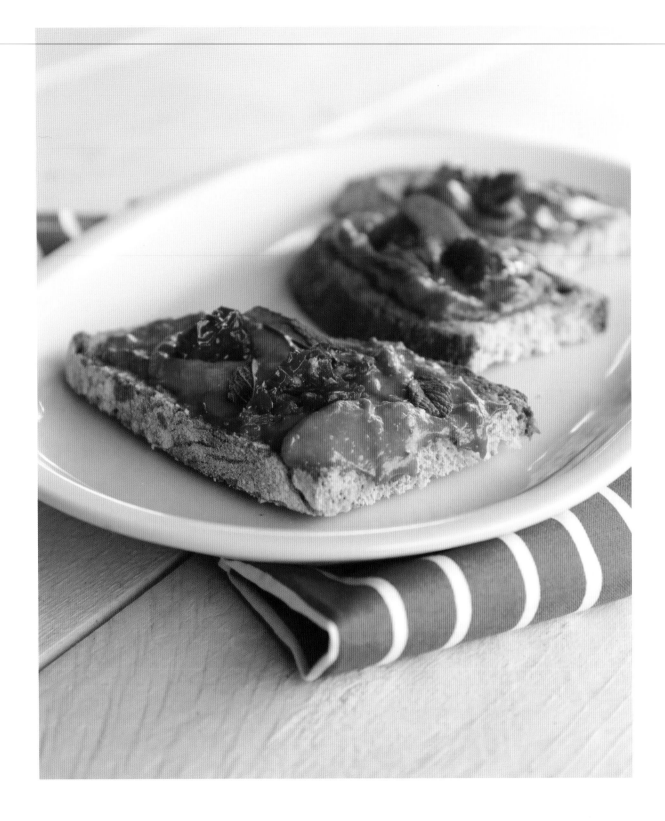

*There are several versions of Sicilian pesto and all have tomatoes as a key ingredient. Of course, summer is the season when tomatoes are juicy and ripe at the right point to give the right flavour to any recipe. The dried fruit is another important key factor. Sicilian pistachios and hazelnuts are ideal for a 100% Sicilian pesto. Failing that, choose good fruit that will ensure a strong flavour and will provide consistency with pesto. Prepare the pesto only a few minutes before serving.*

# CROSTONI WITH SICILIAN PESTO

(CROSTONI CON PESTO SICILIANO)

EF-VEG

*Serves 2*

## INGREDIENTS

- 12 cherry or date tomatoes
- 20 basil leaves
- 100 g (3½ oz) ricotta cheese
- 50 g (1¾ oz) pistachios
- 50 g (1¾ oz) roasted hazelnuts
- 100 g (3½ oz) Parmigiano cheese, grated
- sea salt and pepper
- 150 ml (5 fl oz) extra virgin olive oil
- 2 crusty bread slices

## METHOD

Cut the tomatoes in half and remove the insides.

Using a food processor, process the tomatoes, basil, pistachio, hazelnuts, Parmigiano, salt and pepper. Add the oil and process until creamy.

Spread the pesto sauce over the slices of toast and serve immediately.

*Late spring and summer are the seasons for consuming plenty of vegetables. The fruits of the garden are used to prepare simple dishes, rich in fibre, vitamins and taste.*

*Eggs give the right amount of protein needed to complete a delicious meal, served with chunks of rustic bread.*

# MEDITERRANEAN HERB MIX

(MISTO DI ERBE MEDITERRANEE)

VEG

*Serves 4*

**INGREDIENTS**

- 3 red capsicums (peppers)
- 3 yellow capsicums (peppers)
- 1 onion, roughly chopped
- 2 laurel-bay leaves
- 3 zucchini (courgettes), cut into chunks
- 6 cherry tomatoes, halved
- 2 sage leaves
- 140 ml (4¾ fl oz) extra virgin olive oil, to taste
- pinch of sea salt
- 2 beaten eggs

**METHOD**

Trim the capsicum, removing the stalk, seeds and filaments and cut into pieces.

Hea the olive oil in a frying pan over low heat and add the bay leaves and onion. Cook for 5 minutes. Add a ladle of water, cover and cook for 10 minutes.

Add the capsicum and zucchini and cook for 10 minutes. Add the tomatoes and continue cooking for a further 10 minutes. When cooked, add the salt.

Add the beaten eggs and cook for about 1 minute, so they are still creamy. Serve immediately.

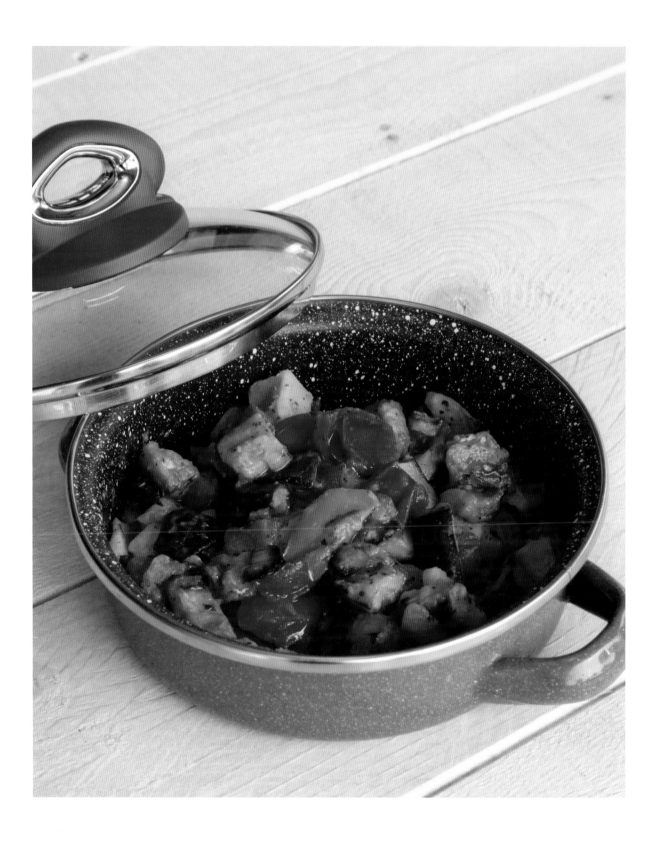

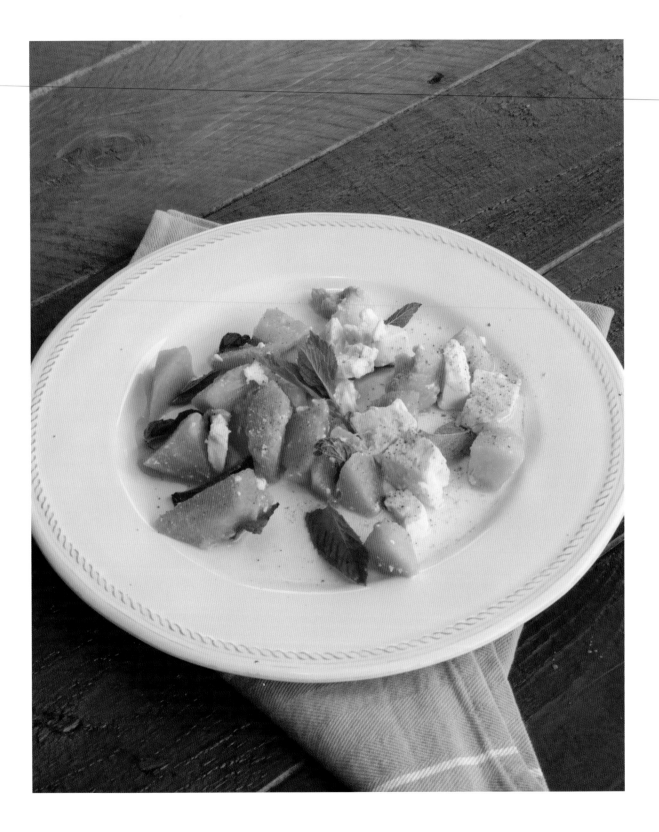

*A salad with a refined taste and elegant colours that encompasses all the beauty of simplicity. Refreshing and tasty, it is ideal to serve as a summer appetizer or side dish.*

# MELON SALAD WITH FETA AND MINT

(INSALATA DI MELONE CON FETA E MENTA)

GF - VEG

*Serves 2-4*

## INGREDIENTS

· 1 melon, cut into cubes
· 250 g (9 oz) feta cheese, cut into cubes
· white pepper, to taste
· sea salt, to taste
· extra virgin olive oil, to taste
· 1 handful mint

## METHOD

Combine the melon and feta. Add the white pepper, sea salt, extra virgin olive oil and mint. Toss gently to combine. Serve immediately or refrigerate until needed.

*Polenta is one of the oldest foods with a strong tradition in northern Italy. Its goodness consists in the quality of the flour and, of course, also in the high quality of the ingredients used to dress it.*

*Usually, the cheeses are the ideal match. Polenta with cheese is one of my beloved foods, especially when I spend a few days in the beautiful mountains of Valle D'Aosta. There, in front of a fireplace, I always find the ideal atmosphere to enjoy a dish as simple and delicious as this one.*

*This is the perfect dish to serve for an informal brunch on a chilly day. Simple high-quality ingredients make this recipe ideal.*

# POLENTA WITH LEEKS AND CHEESE

(POLENTA CON PORRI E FORMAGGIO)

EF-VEG

*Serves 4*

### INGREDIENTS

· 400 g (14 oz) pre-cooked polenta
· 2 leeks, cut into rounds
· 100 ml (3½ fl oz) warm water
· pinch of sea salt

· 150 g (5½ oz) Fontina cheese, cut into cubes
· 50 g (1¾ oz) Parmigiano, grated
· extra virgin olive oil, to taste

### METHOD

Boil 1,5 litres (52 fl oz) of salted water over medium heat. Add the polenta and stir to avoid the formation of lumps. Cook for about 8–10 minutes, or according to the directions on the packaging (traditional polenta has a very long cooking time. About 50 minutes).

Sauté the leeks with some olive oil in a pan over medium heat. Add the water and salt and cook, lid on, for about 10 minutes.

Add the Fontina and Parmigiano to the hot polenta and mix until they have melted. Add the leeks and serve warm with a drizzle of olive oil.

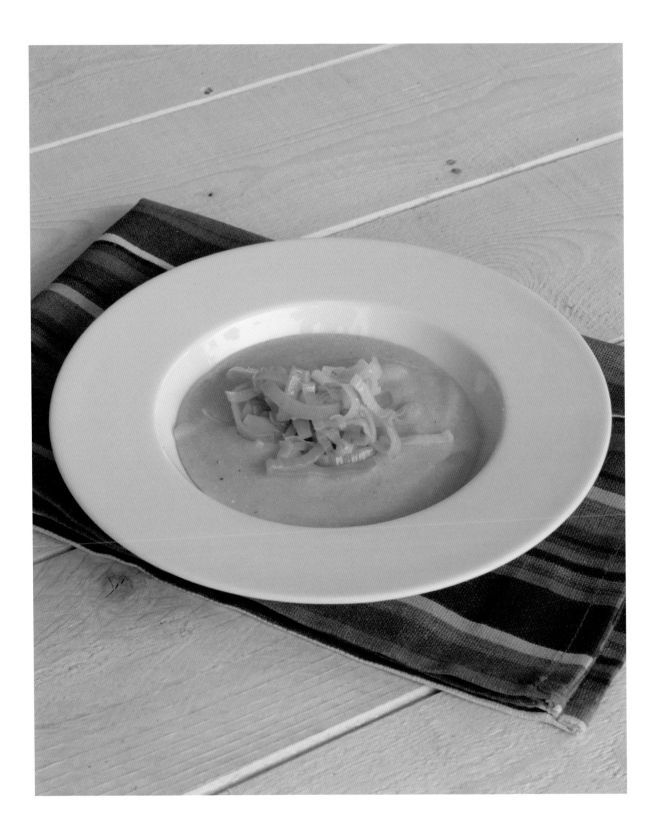

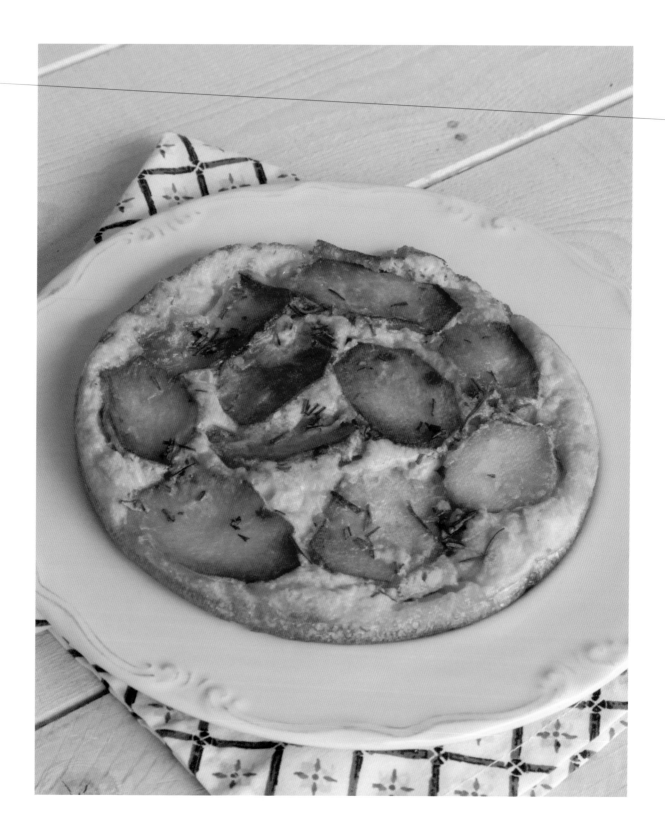

*Frittata is a classic of Italian cuisine. It is one of the first dishes that Italians learn to cook. The reason probably stems from being a dish easy to perform.*

*It can be eaten either hot or cold. It is delicious served still warm. Frittata is ideal for a brunch or as a cold appetizer, cut into cubes.*

*I prepare the frittata just baked. This type of cooking is much healthier and the taste is guaranteed.*

# POTATO FRITTATA WITH ROSEMARY

(FRITTATA DI PATATE CON ROSMARINO)

VEG

*Serves 4*

## INGREDIENTS

- 2 onions
- 500 g (1 lb 2 oz) potatoes, peeled and roughly chopped
- 1 handful chopped rosemary
- 5 tablespoons grated Parmigiano cheese
- 2 tablespoons grated Pecorino cheese
- 4 large eggs
- 3 tablespoons milk
- extra virgin olive oil, to taste
- pinch of sea salt and pepper

## METHOD

Peel and finely chop the onions, sauté for 4-5 minutes on low heat in a saucepan with 5 tablespoons of oil. Add 1 ladle of hot water, salt and cover, continuing cooking for 15 minutes, adding more hot water, if necessary.

Boil the potatoes in a saucepan full of salted water for 15 minutes. Drain. Add the potatoes to a non-stick frying pan over medium heat with a little oil and the chopped rosemary. Add the cooked onions, cook for a few minutes and leave to cool.

Preheat the oven to 180°C (350°F/Gas 4). Line a baking tin with baking paper.

Beat the eggs in a bowl and add the Parmigiano, Pecorino, milk, a pinch of salt and stir. Add the potatoes and onions and mix well.

Pour the mixture into a baking tin and bake for 15 minutes.

*If you have a few good ingredients in the pantry and if you have little time, this recipe is ideal.*
*With garden vegetables and the excellent, creamy Robiola, I love to prepare this recipe, perfect for a brunch with friends, mid-morning snack or a light dinner.*

# PUFF PASTRY WITH GRILLED EGGPLANT, TOMATOES AND PEPPER SAUCE

(SFOGLIA CON MELANZANE GRIGLIATE, SALSA DI POMODORO E PEPERONI)

VEG

*Serves 4*

## INGREDIENTS

- 250 g (9 oz) organic puff pastry, palm oil free
- 1 eggplant (aubergine), thinly sliced lengthways
- 1 red chilli
- 150 g (5½ oz) tomato paste (concentrated purée)
- 1 handful basil
- pinch of sea salt
- 4 tablespoons extra virgin olive oil
- 100 g (3½ oz) Robiola cheese
- 1 handful or rocket (arugula) or valerian

## METHOD

Preheat the oven to 180°C (350°F/Gas 4). Line a 35cm round baking tray with baking paper.

Roll out the pastry into the tray, prick and bake for 15 minutes.

Washed, cut the eggplant and grilled.

Grill the eggplant on a barbecue chargrill plate or in a chargrill pan.

Using a blender or food processor, process the chilli pepper with the tomato sauce, basil, salt and oil.

Pour the sauce on the puff pastry, place on top of the eggplant and bake for 10 minutes.

Once baked, add the Robiola, rocket (arugula) or valerian.

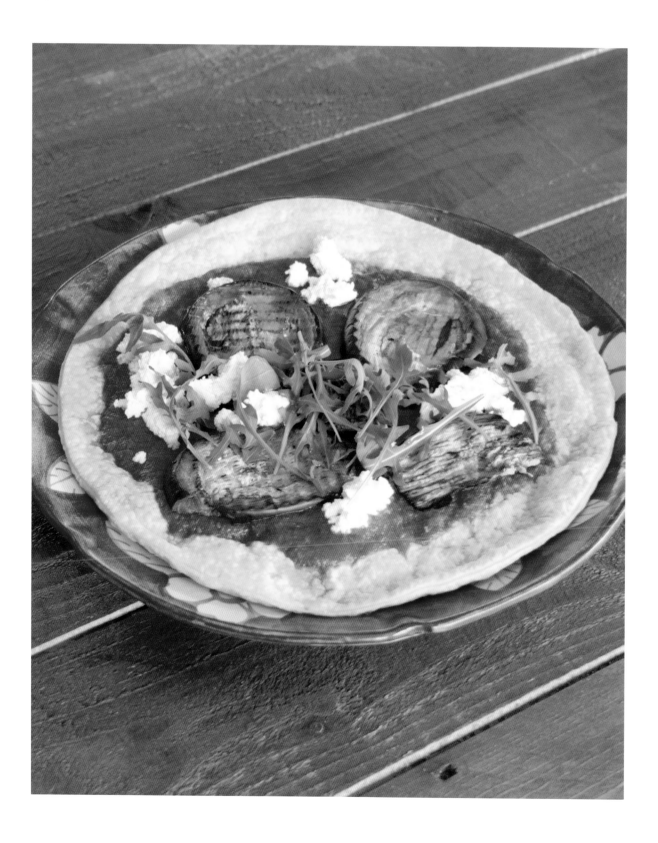

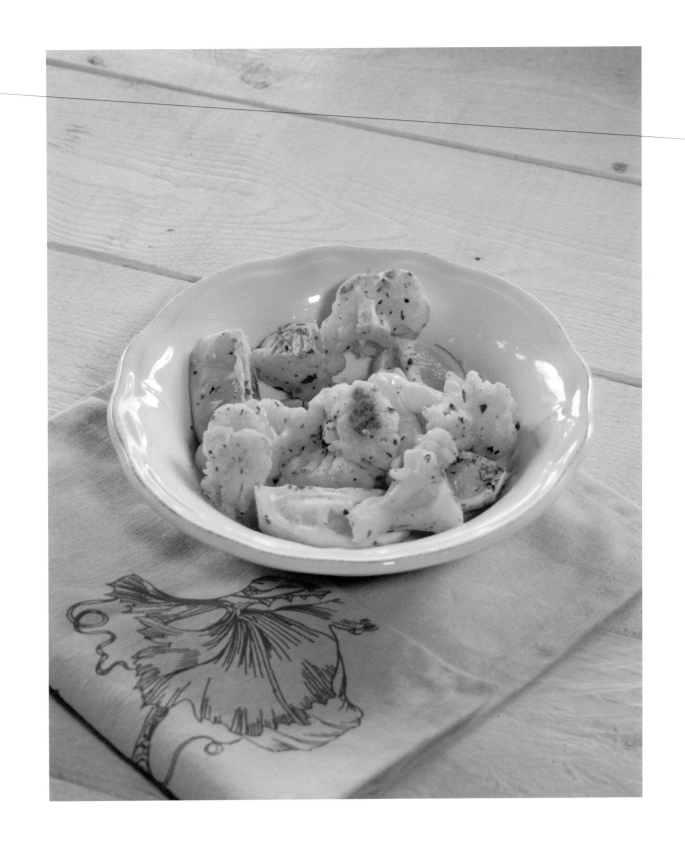

*I usually serve roasted cauliflower with rustic bread, dried fruit and vegetable cutlets (seitan or tofu). The aroma and texture are wonderful. A very tasty way to enjoy vegetables—even for those who are usually reluctant.*

# ROASTED CAULIFLOWER

(CAVOLFIORI AL FORNO)

GF-V

*Serves 4*

**INGREDIENTS**

- 300 g (10½ oz) cauliflower florets
- pinch of sea salt
- zest of 1 lemon, roughly chopped
- extra virgin olive oil, to taste
- white pepper, to taste

**METHOD**

Preheat the oven to 180°C (350°F/Gas 4). Lightly grease a roasting tin and line with baking paper. Boil the cauliflower florets in a saucepan filled with salted water for 10–15 minutes or until al dente. Add the cauliflower florets, lemon zest, extra virgin olive oil and pepper to the tin and toss to coat. Place the roasting tin on the top shelf of the oven and cook for about 25 minutes.

*I really love spinach and cultivate it in my garden. Fresh and organic spinach are so tender that they require very little cooking. Their scent is delicious and it is also enhanced by simple recipes like this.*

*Perfect for a snack, brunch or as an appetizer, accompanied by soft cheeses. Ideal freshly baked, they can also be kept in an airtight container for 3–4 days.*

# SPINACH AND LEMON SAVOURY CAKES

(TORTINE DI SPINACI CON LIMONE)

VEG

*Makes 8–10*

## INGREDIENTS

- 300 g (10½ oz) baby English spinach
- pinch of sea salt
- pepper, to taste
- 1 large egg
- zest and lemon juice
- 4 tablespoons milk (or rice milk)

- 50 ml (1¾ fl oz) extra virgin olive oil
- 300 g (10½ oz) wholemeal (whole-wheat) wheat flour, sifted
- 15 g (½ oz) organic baking powder (for savoury cakes)

## METHOD

Preheat the oven to 180°C (350°F/Gas 4). Lightly grease ten muffin holes.

Trim the spinach, discarding the stems and thick leaves. Put the spinach in a large pot over medium heat and cook for 8–10 minutes. Halfway through cooking, add a pinch of salt and pepper to taste.

Lightly beat the egg in a bowl with the salt, grated zest, lemon juice and oil. Add the spinach and stir in the flour sifted with the baking powder. Stir to combine well.

Pour the mixture into the muffin holes. Bake for 15–20 minutes, or until lightly golden. Leave to cool in the tin for 5 minutes, then turn out onto a wire rack to cool.

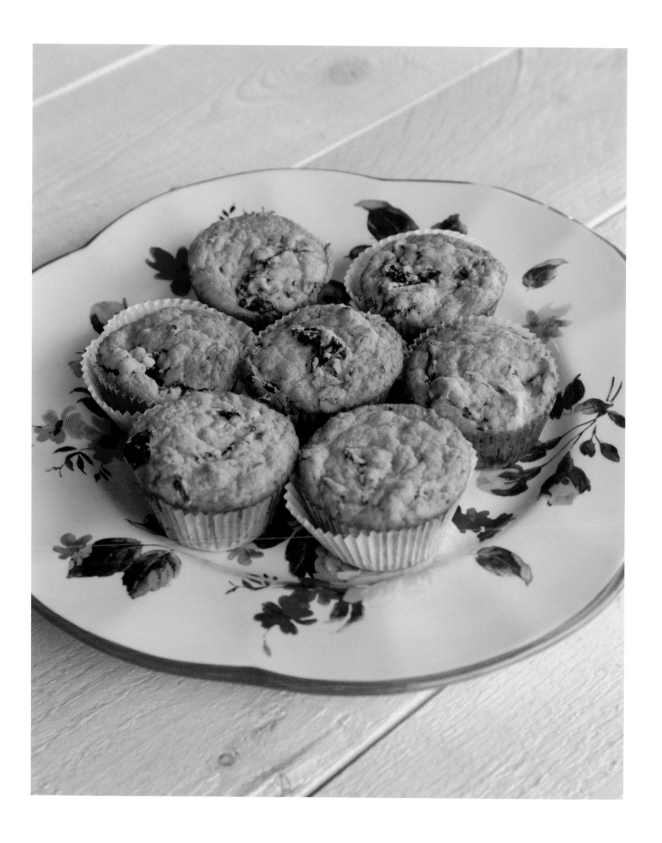

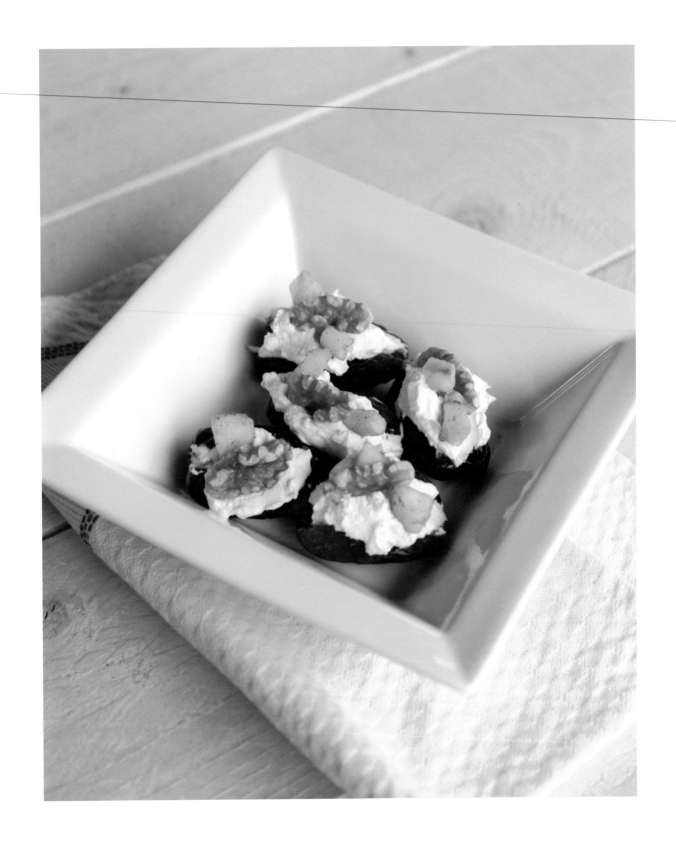

*This is a classic appetizer at Christmas time when the dates (and dried fruit in general) are the protagonists at the Italian table. Dates are delicious, and are an alternative to white sugar. They are also high in fiber, iron, vitamins and minerals. Dates are a natural anti-inflammatory, suitable for colds and respiratory irritation. Ricotta is a perfect match here because of its delicate flavour.*

# STUFFED DATES

(DATTERI RIPIENI)

EG-VEG

*Serves 6-8*

## INGREDIENTS

- 2 pears (1 if large), peeled and diced
- juice of 1 lemon
- 100 g (3½ oz) ricotta cheese
- pinch of ground cinnamon

- 1 tablespoon date nectar (or raw honey)
- 10 Medjoul dates
- 50 g (1¾ oz) chopped walnuts

## METHOD

Place the diced pear in a bowl and drizzle with lemon juice to prevent blackening.
Combine the ricotta, cinnamon and the juice of the dates in a bowl. Stir until the mixture is creamy.
Halve the dates, remove the core with a spoon and stuff with the ricotta mixture.
Garnish with the diced pears and walnuts. Serve immediately.

*Filled tomatoes filled are a classic Italian antipasti.*
*Creamy tofu (or Silk tofu), ~~combined with the freshness of basil and wild fennel~~, really makes this delicious recipe special. If you do not like tofu you can replace it with a vegan cheese.*
*For a vegetarian alternative you can make this recipe with soft cheese, such as Robiola or Crescenza.*

# TOMATOES FILLED WITH TOFU, WILD FENNEL AND PINE NUTS

(POMODORI CON TOFU SETA, FINOCCHIETTO SELVATICO E PINOLI)

DF- GF-V

### Serves 4

**INGREDIENTS**

· 4 firm fresh tomatoes (in season)
· 200 g (7 oz) silken tofu
· pinch of sea salt
· pepper, to taste

· 1 tablespoon extra virgin olive oil
· 6 basil leaves
· 1 handful wild fennel
· 1 tablespoon roasted pine nuts

**METHOD**

Wash the tomatoes, cut the tops off and remove the seeds and pulp using a small knife or a spoon.
Knead the tofu with a generous pinch of salt, pepper and 1 tablespoon of oil.
Tear the basil leaves and wild fennel using your hands and add to the tofu.
Fill the tomatoes with the creamy tofu mixture, decorate with toasted pine nuts and serve.

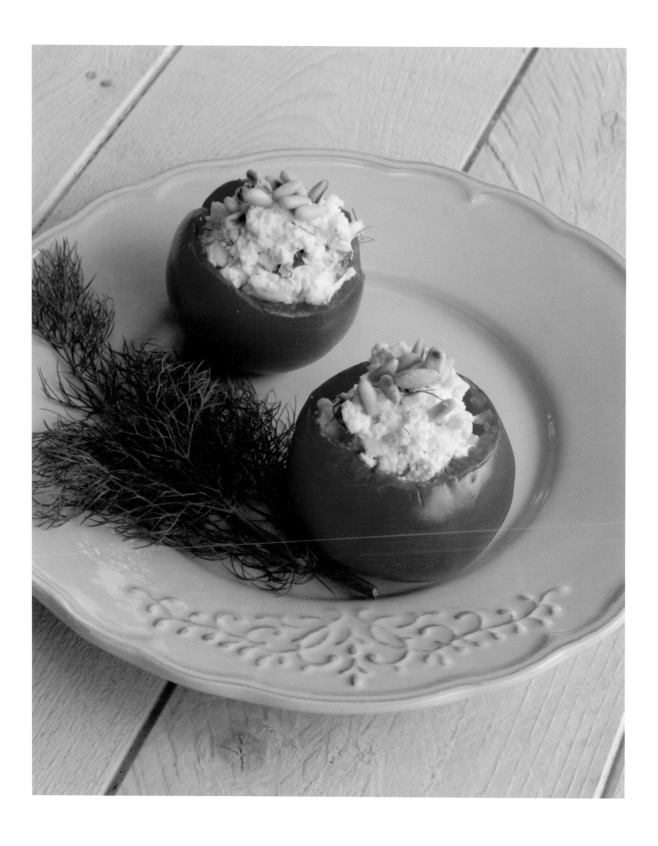

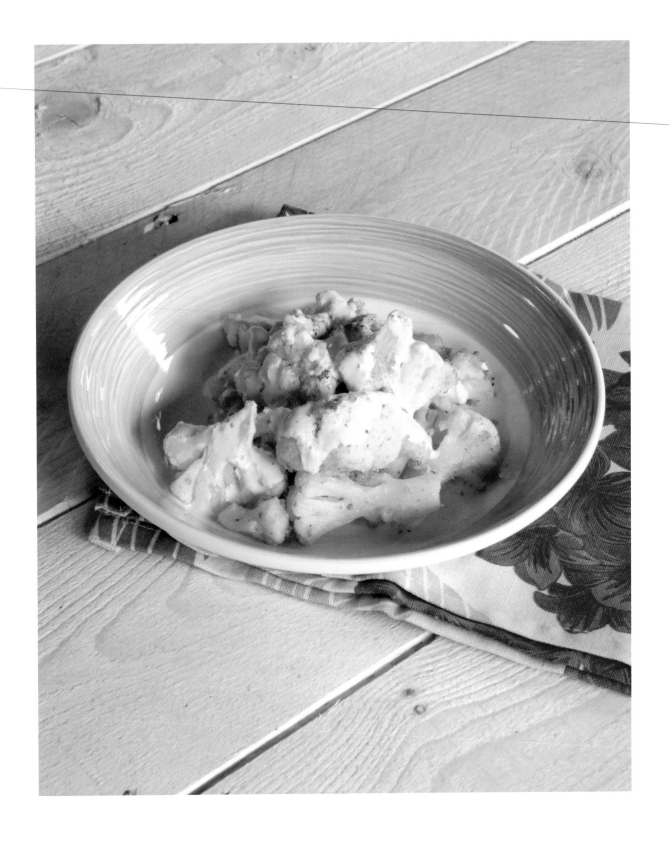

*I love this dish because is very easy to make and is completely vegan. In addition, it is a true winter comfort food and one of my favourites. Gluten-free rice sauce (or béchamel), so light and delicious, is the key of the recipe. Of course, you can replace cauliflower with broccoli or put them together for a concentration of vitamin C, beta-carotene and antioxidants.*

# WHITE CAULIFLOWER GRATIN

(GRATIN DI CAVOLFIORI BIANCHI)

GF-V

### Serves 2

## INGREDIENTS

- 300 g (10½ oz) cauliflower florets
- 250 ml (9 fl oz) rice milk
- 50 g (1¾ oz) almond flour
- 2 tablespoons brown rice flour, sifted
- 1 teaspoon nutmeg

- pepper, to taste
- extra virgin olive oil, to taste
- gluten-free breadcrumbs, to taste
- sea salt, to taste

## METHOD

Blanch the cauliflower florets in a pot with salted water over medium heat for about 15–20 minutes. Drain and set aside until needed.

Preheat the oven to 180°C (350°F/Gas 4). Lightly grease a baking tin.

In a separate saucepan, boil the rice milk over medium heat. Reduce the heat and add the almond flour, rice flour, nutmeg and pepper and stir with a whisk until mixture has a thick consistency.

Place the cauliflower in the baking tin, coat with the sauce, sprinkle with breadcrumbs and bake for 15 minutes. Serve warm.

*When zucchini (courgettes) hit the farmer's market, you know summer has arrived. I love my zucchini from the garden and, when in season, I eat them every day.*

*Savoury cakes are my favourite because they lend themselves to so many situations and, at times they are perfect for a light but nutritious lunch. This luscious rustic savoury cake is perfect freshly baked or the day after.*

# ZUCCHINI CAKE

GF-VEG

### Serves 4

## INGREDIENTS

- 1 spring onion (scallion), finely sliced
- 4 zucchini (courgettes), grated
- 3 eggs
- pinch of sea salt
- 100 g (3¹/₂ oz) Fontina (or Taleggio) cheese, cut into cubes
- 120 ml (4 fl oz) extra virgin olive oil
- 300 g (10¹/₂ oz) brown rice flour, sifted
- 1 tablespoon organic baking powder
- 75 ml (2¹/₄ fl oz) organic cow milk
- 100 g (3¹/₂ oz) feta cheese, crumbled
- 1 handful basil leaves, torn

## METHOD

Preheat the oven to 180°C (350°F/Gas 4). Lightly grease a 35 cm square or round tin.

In a frying pan over medium heat, sauté the spring onion and zucchini with 2 tablespoons of the olive oil.

Beat the eggs with a pinch of salt, add the cheese and the remaining oil. Add the flour, baking powder and milk and stir to combine.

Add the zucchini mixture, feta and basil. Pour the mixture into a mold lined with baking paper and bake for 35-40 minutes. Leave to cool in the tin for 5 minutes before transferring to a wire rack to cool.

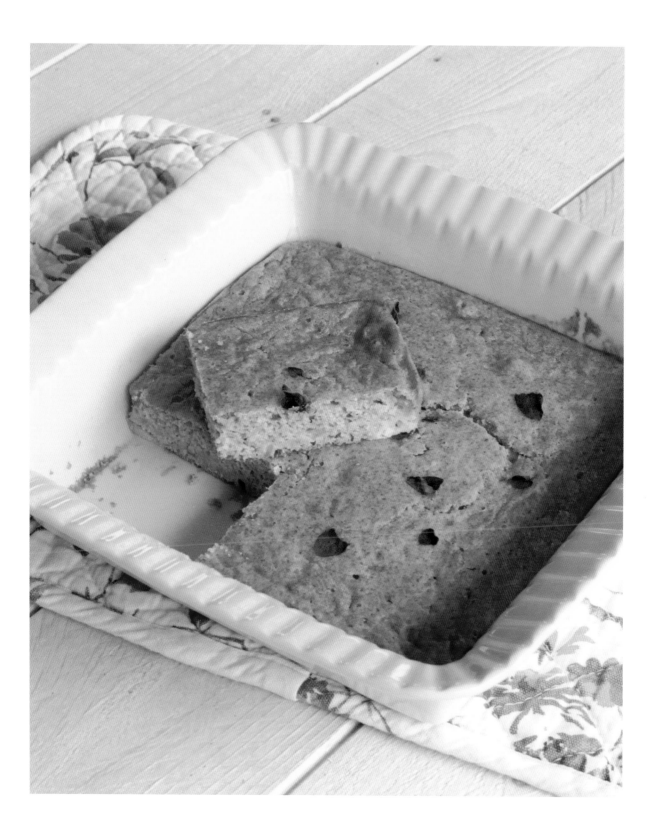

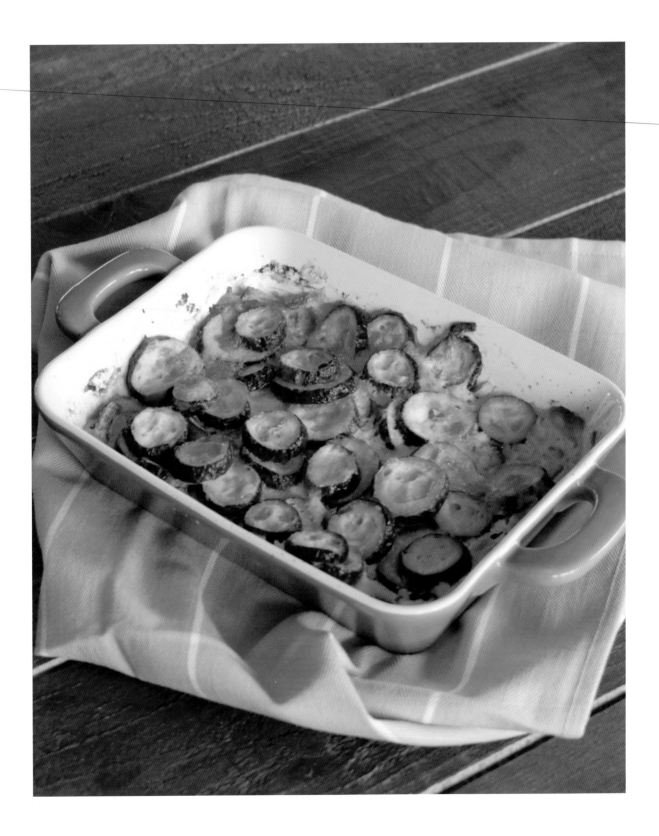

*Baked zucchini (courgettes) is a tasty and healthy solution to consume seasonal vegetables with various combinations of ingredients.*

*Zucchini goes perfectly with cheese. Parmigiano and Provola are two of the most renowned Italian specialty cheeses—perfect for this recipe. You can replace them with high-quality local cheeses.*

# ZUCCHINI GRATIN

### (GRATIN DI ZUCCHINE)

VEG

*Serves 4*

### INGREDIENTS
- 2 onions, roughly chopped
- 8 zucchini (courgettes), cut into slices
- 2 large eggs
- 120 ml (4 fl oz) cows milk
- 50 g (2 oz) grated Parmigiano cheese
- 150 g (5¹/₂ oz) Provola cheese, cut into cubes
- extra virgin olive oil, to taste

### METHOD
Sauté the onions with some olive oil in a frying pan over low heat for 5 minutes. Add 1 tablespoon of water, cover and cook for 5 minutes. Add the zucchini and cook for a further 10 minutes, adding salt halfway through cooking.

Preheat the oven to 180°C (350°F/Gas 4). Lightly grease a baking tin.

Beat the eggs with the milk and Parmigiano. Add the zucchini to the baking tin. Pour the cheese and bake for 20 minutes.

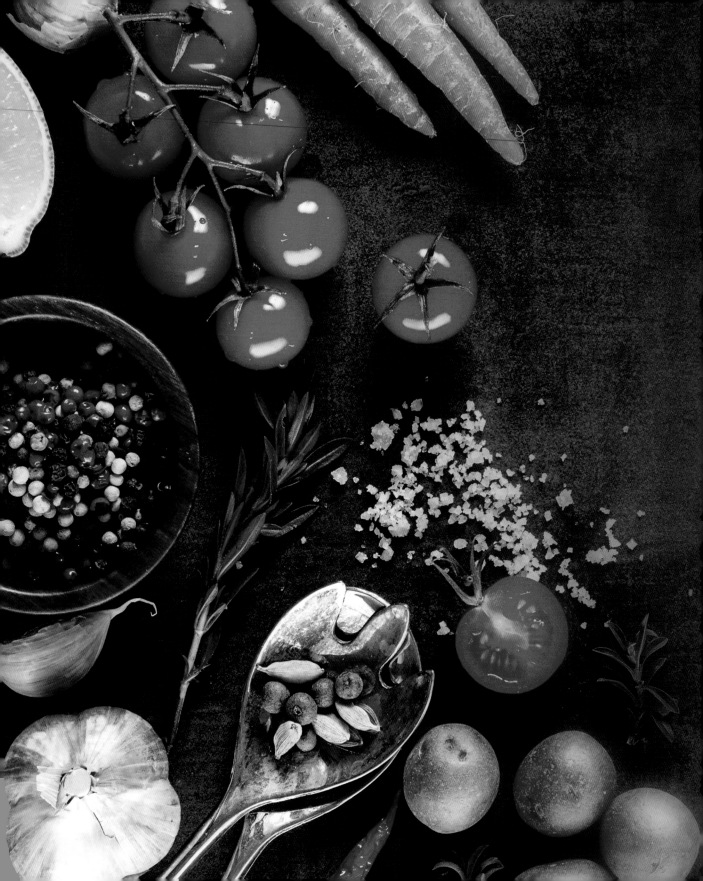

# VEGETABLES

Italian cuisine offers dishes rich in vegetables. Italians love seasonal vegetables. We usually prefer to buy them from the local markets, where goods have fair prices and the quality of products is high. The secret lies in this small but important trick.

Eating healthily means knowing what we put on the plate. Today this step is essential.

The vegetables in supermarkets are controlled and offer some guarantees. But they all look the same. What's tasty about a zucchini, eggplant and tomato available all year round? Is it really worth putting this kind of vegetable, which could possibly be rich in pesticides, on our plate?

Those who cultivate their own vegetable garden, or those who buy from local producers, know that vegetables grown without pesticides (or with a reduced content of pesticides) have a much more normal size and a unique flavour. This is priceless.

Learn to appreciate the beauty of nature, and let's dedicate ourselves to the knowledge of what we eat, without throwing in the shopping cart vegetables only based on beauty. Let us nourish ourselves with awareness and choose seasonality. Each season has so many vegetables. We are spoiled for choice.

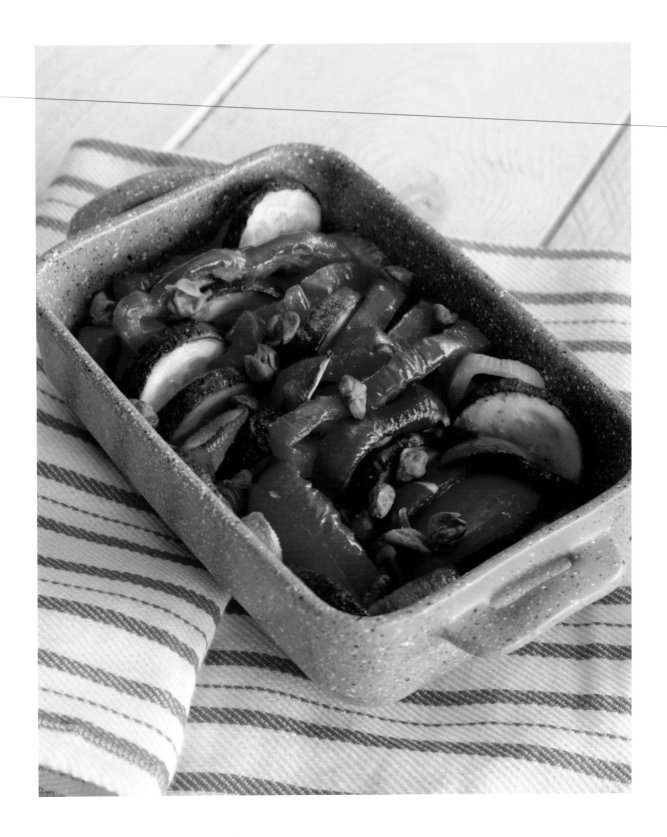

*Summer vegetables are among the most popular. Their bright colours and their versatility makes them ideal for many preparations.*

*I love to cook these vegetables in the oven. They are delicious freshly baked but are also perfect the next day, seasoned with a little extra virgin olive oil.*

# BAKED VEGETABLES

(VERDURE AL FORNO)

V

*Serves 2- 4*

## INGREDIENTS

- 2 eggplant (aubergines), cut into rounds
- 2 red capsicum (pepper)
- 3 zucchini (courgettes), cut into rounds
- 2 red onions, sliced
- 2 tomatoes, sliced

- extra virgin olive oil, to taste
- pinch of sea salt
- white pepper, to taste
- 1 tablespoon dry oregano
- 2 tablespoons de-salted capers

## METHOD

Place the eggplant in a bowl. Add the water and salt and cover with a plate, leaving it to sit for about 30 minutes. Rinse and dry the eggplants.

Preheat the oven to 180°C (350°F/Gas 4). Lightly grease a baking tin.

Discard the stems, seeds and filaments of the capsicums and roughly chop.

Place the vegetables in the baking tin, add extra virgin olive oil, a pinch of salt and pepper and the oregano.

Roast in the oven for about 30–35 minutes. Serve the vegetables warm, garnished with de-salted capers.

*Barley is one of the ideal foods in the cold months. Widely used in northern Italy (together with buckwheat), it is rich in iron and vitamin C and does not raise the levels of glucose in the blood.*
*If consumed with winter vegetables, it becomes a tasty complete dish, to be eaten several times a week.*

# BARLEY WITH WINTER VEGETABLES

(ORZO CON VERDURE INVERNALI)

V

*Serves 4*

## INGREDIENTS

- 300 g (10½ oz) barley
- 500 ml (17 fl oz) water
- sea salt, to taste
- 6 broccoli florets
- 2 carrots, sliced
- 1 spring onion

- 3 tablespoons extra virgin olive oil
- 1 garlic clove
- zest of 1 lemon
- 2 eggs
- 1 tablespoon dried oregano
- pinch of sea salt

## METHOD

Rinse the barley and drain. In a heavy-based pot, toast the barley for 5 minutes. Add the water and a pinch of salt. Bring to the boil and cook, covered with a lid, for about 25–30 minutes.

Cut the broccoli florets in two.

Heat 3 tablespoons of extra virgin olive oil in a large frying pan over medium heat. Add the garlic and lemon zest and sauté until lightly browned.

Add the vegetables and cook until *al dente*, so that the colour is still bright.

Beat the eggs, season with oregano, a pinch of salt and scramble in a saucepan with a some oil over medium heat.

Add the barley to the vegetables and mix. Add the eggs, some oil and serve hot.

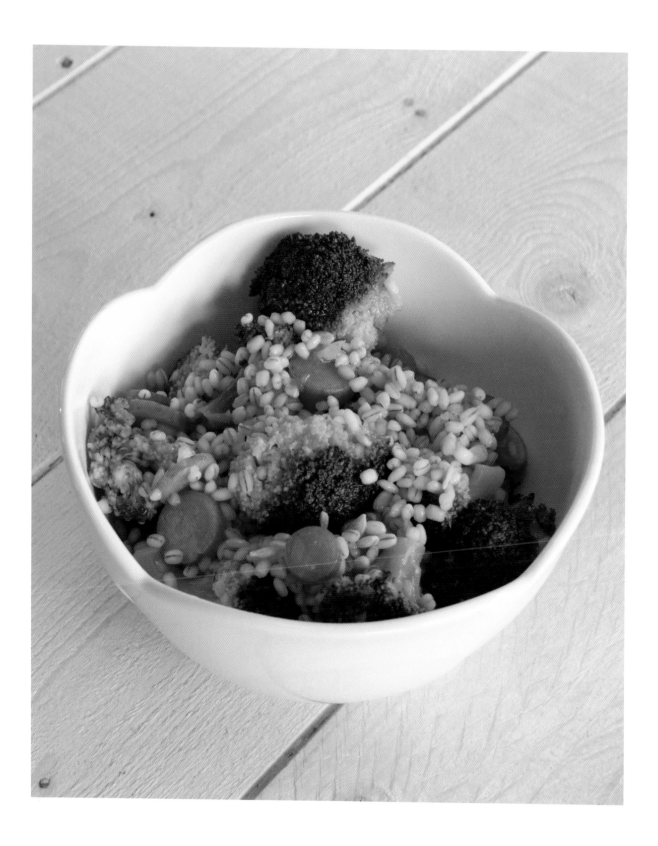

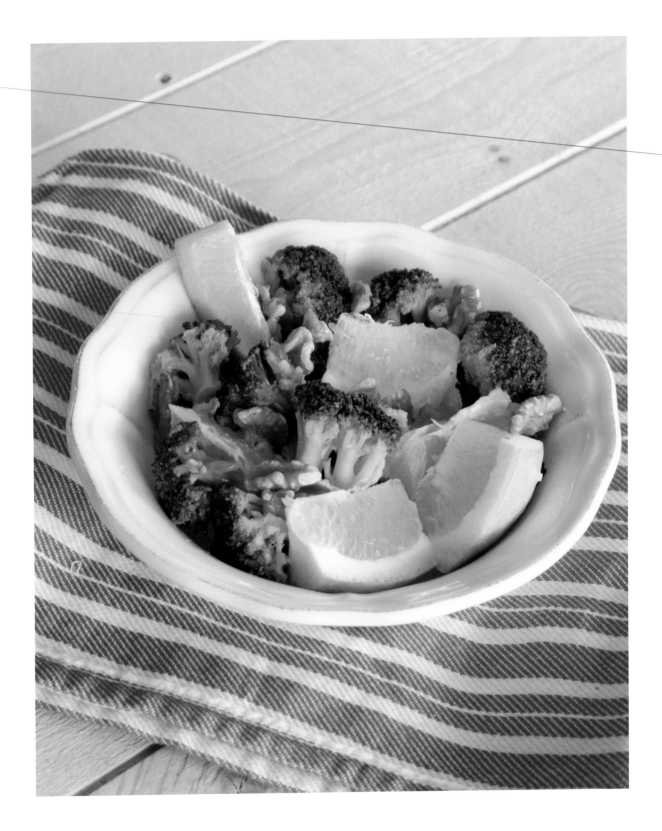

*Broccoli is one of the winter vegetables I love most. I like to cook it in various ways and this salad is one of my favourites. I consider it a real cure against winter colds. Broccoli and lemon are rich in vitamin C.*
*You can replace the walnuts with other nuts. The white wine can be omitted, although it makes a difference.*

# BROCCOLI WITH LEMON AND WALNUTS

(BROCCOLI CON LIMONE E NOCI)

GF-V

### Serves 2

## INGREDIENTS

- 400 g (14 oz) broccoli florets
- 1 garlic clove
- 1 onion, chopped
- pinch of sea salt
- white pepper, to taste
- 100 ml (3$^1$/$_2$ oz) white wine
- 50 ml (1$^3$/$_4$ fl oz) water
- extra virgin olive oil, to taste
- 1 tablespoon walnuts
- 1 lemon

## METHOD

Place the broccoli florets in a saucepan with the garlic, onion, salt, pepper, wine, water and extra virgin olive oil.

Bring to the boil and cook for 20–25 minutes, depending on the desired consistency.

Serve with chopped walnuts and lemon slices.

*This beautiful dish is an ode to joy. The recipe is complete with all the necessary nutrients and can be modified according to your tastes. Rice can be replaced with farro, buckwheat or other grains, vegetables can be rotated according to the season and pumpkin seeds and almonds can be replaced with pistachios, walnuts, hazelnuts or cashews.*

# BROWN RICE WITH RADICCHIO, PUMPKIN AND PUMPKIN SEEDS

(RISO INTEGRALE CON RADICCHIO, ZUCCA E SEMI DI ZUCCA)

GF-V

*Serves 4*

### INGREDIENTS

- 300 g (10¹/₂ oz) brown rice
- 200 g (7 oz) pumpkin (winter squash), cut into cubes
- 2 spring onions (scallions), thinly sliced
- 2 radicchio, chopped
- 1 tablespoon toasted white almonds
- 1 tablespoon pumpkin seeds
- extra virgin olive oil, to taste
- pinch of sea salt

### METHOD

Rinse the rice and cook in a pot filled with salted water for about 30–35 minutes. Drain and season with olive oil and a pinch of salt.

Heat 1 tablespoon of oil in a frying pan over medium heat. Add the pumpkin and spring onions. Add the radicchio and cook for 3–4 minutes. Add a pinch of salt during cooking.

In a salad bowl, add the rice, top with the vegetables and serve with toasted white almonds and pumpkin seeds.

*This dish often appears on my summer table. A concentration of colours, flavours, fragrances and vitamins. But this is not just a tomato salad. It is a tribute to the culinary wonders of Southern Italy. The Sicilian cherry tomatoes are simply unique. In the summer, my garden is full of these little gems that I eat raw, seasoned in different ways. Sicilian capers and onion of Tropea make a difference in flavour and also in appearance.*

# TOMATOES WITH CAPERS

(POMODORINI CANDITI CON CAPPERI)

EF-V

*Serves 2*

**INGREDIENTS**

- 400 g (14 oz) cherry tomatoes, halved
- 1 tablespoon raw coconut sugar, to taste
- pinch of sea salt
- 1 garlic clove, chopped
- 1 tablespoon oregano
- 1 thyme sprig
- extra virgin olive oil, to taste
- 1 red onion, sliced
- 1 tablespoon salted capers

**METHOD**

Preheat the oven to 180°C (350°F/Gas 4). Lightly grease and line a baking tray with baking paper.

Arrange the tomatoes on the tray. Sprinkle with sugar and salt and cook for 1 hour 30 minutes.

Transfer the tomatoes to a large bowl and add the garlic, oregano, thyme and olive oil and mix. Set aside for 30 minutes.

Add the onion and capers to the tomatoes. Remove the garlic, stir and serve.

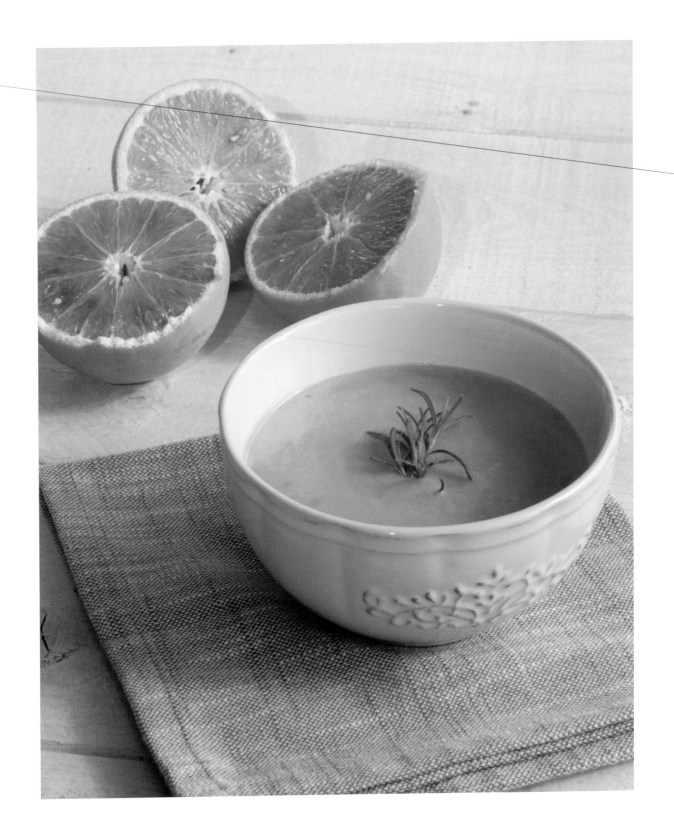

*This recipe is a concentration of vitamin C, perfect for the winter. During the cold season, oranges are the heroes of the Sicilian table. Sicilian blood oranges are reported to have nutritional properties superior to traditional oranges. Among the many useful substances for the prevention of various diseases, there are the anthocyanins, natural pigments which give the red oranges all their colour and the unique flavour. They are key to this delicious dish. You can replace them with traditional oranges.*

# CARROT AND RED ORANGE SOUP

(CREMA DI CAROTE E ARANCE ROSSE)

GF-V

*Serves 4*

## INGREDIENTS

- 300 g (10$^1$/$_2$ oz) carrots, pee
- 1 onion, finely chopped
- 3 tablespoons red oranges juice
- 3 tablespoons lemon juice
- 250 ml (9 fl oz) water
- 100 ml (3$^1$/$_2$ oz) organic fresh cream (or rice

cream palm oil free)
- extra virgin olive oil, to taste
- pinch of salt
- 1 rosemary sprig
- white pepper, to taste

## METHOD

Steam the carrots until they are soft.

Heat 1 tablespoon of olive oil in a frying pan over medium heat. Add the onion and cook for a few minutes. Add the carrots, crushing them with a fork.

Add the citrus juice and cook for about 15 minutes over low heat. Gradually add the water (if necessary, add more water). Whisk the mixture.

Add the cream and season with salt, rosemary and sprinkle with white pepper.

*I love velvety soups. They are the main course of my weekly supper club with my friends. In spring, asparagus soup is never missing in my table. Unfortunately, the asparagus season is very short but, because of that, they are a little treasure to consume as much as possible to reap all the benefits.*

# CREAMY ASPARAGUS SOUP

(VELLUTATA DI ASPARAGI)

GF-V

*Serves 2*

## INGREDIENTS

· 300 g (10¹⁄₂ oz) asparagus
· 2 spring onions (scallions), diced
· sea salt, to taste

· extra virgin olive oil, to taste
· 1 mint sprig

## METHOD

With a knife remove the film layer that covers the white part of the asparagus. Wash them. Cut off the terminal.

Cook the asparagus in a pot filled with salted water for 15–20 minutes (time cooking varies according to the size of the asparagus).

Once cooked, purée the asparagus in a blender, adding 2 tablespoons of olive oil and, if necessary, water to taste.

Season with a drizzle of extra virgin olive oil and a sprig of mint. Serve immediately.

*If possible, buy potatoes from local producers. Their taste and freshness will surprise you.*
*The flavour of this recipe becomes even more special with the feta and a few drops of balsamic vinegar.*

# POTATO AND ONION SALAD

(INSALATA DI PATATE E CIPOLLE ROSSE)

EF-VEG

*Serves 2*

**INGREDIENTS**

- 4 potatoes
- 1 flat-leaf (Italian) parsley sprig, chopped
- 3 red onions
- 100 g (3½ oz) feta cheese
- balsamic vinegar, to taste
- extra virgin olive oil, to taste
- pinch of sea salt

**METHOD**

Boil the potatoes in salted water for about 30 minutes (depending on size of potatoes).
Soak the onion in water until ready to serve.
Drain the potatoes, leave to cool, then peel and cut into chunks.
Combine the potatoes, parsley, onions and feta in a bowl. Season with extra virgin olive oil and salt.
  Serve immediately.

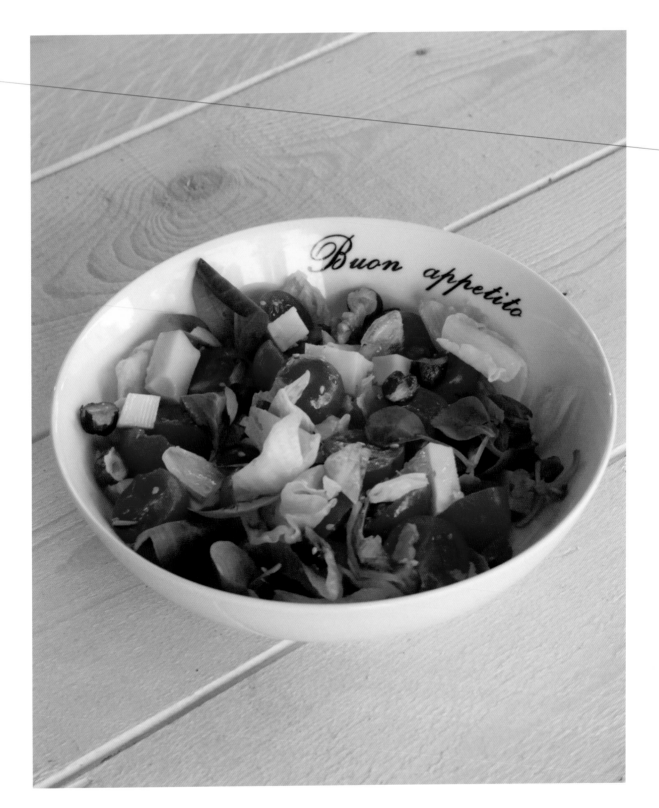

Salads can become a substantial main dish—rich in vitamins, minerals and proteins. The key is to select seasonal vegetables, preferably organic.

In this recipe I have used cos (romaine) lettuce and valerian, both rich in vitamin C, antioxidants, iron, calcium, magnesium and potassium.

I also added a generous handful of Sicilian toasted hazelnuts. Hazelnuts have important nutritional properties. They contain monounsaturated fats (the "good fats"), vitamins E and K, minerals such as potassium, calcium and phosphorus.

# CRUNCHY SUMMER SALAD

(INSALATA ESTIVA CROCCANTE)

GF - VEG

*Serves 2*

## INGREDIENTS

· 6 cos (romaine) lettuce leaves
· 1 generous handful valerian leaves
· 10–15 cherry tomatoes, cut in half
· 2 tablespoons chopped toasted hazelnuts
· 100 g (3½ oz) semi-hard cheese, cut into cubes
  (or feta, or cherry mozzarella to your liking)
· 2 tablespoons Modena balsamic vinegar
· 4–5 tablespoons extra virgin olive oil
· pinch of sea salt
· pepper, to taste

## METHOD

Place all the vegetables in a large bowl. Add the chopped hazelnuts and cheese.

In another bowl, add the balsamic vinegar, extra virgin olive oil, pinch of sea salt and pepper to taste. Emulsify with a fork and leave for 5 minutes.

Add the dressing to the salad. Mix well and let stand in refrigerator for 30 minutes before serving.

Serve with slices of rustic bread, if you like.

*Summer eggplants (aubergines) are a triumph and favourite ingredient of Italian cuisine. Fried or baked, there are dozens of recipes that you can prepare while they are in season.*

*This is a very simple idea for a delicious side dish but is also an excellent solution for filling sandwiches. Baked and breaded, the eggplant is beautiful when served with bright tomatoes and fresh basil.*

# EGGPLANT CUTLETS

### (COTOLETTE DI MELANZANE)

DF

### *Makes about 15 cutlets*

**INGREDIENTS**

- 2 large organic eggplants (aubergines), sliced
- pinch of sea salt
- 100 g ($3^1/_2$ oz) brown rice flour
- 1 large egg
- 100 g ($3^1/_2$ oz) breadcrumbs
- extra virgin olive oil, to taste

**METHOD**

Soak the eggplant in water for 30 minutes.

Preheat the oven to 180°C (350°F/Gas 4). Line a baking tray with baking paper.

In three separate dishes, place the flour, breadcrumbs and eggs.

Drain the eggplants and pat dry with paper towel. Dip each eggplant slice in the flour, then the eggs and then in the breadcrumbs.

Arrange the eggplant on the baking tray. Bake for 25 minutes, or until golden.

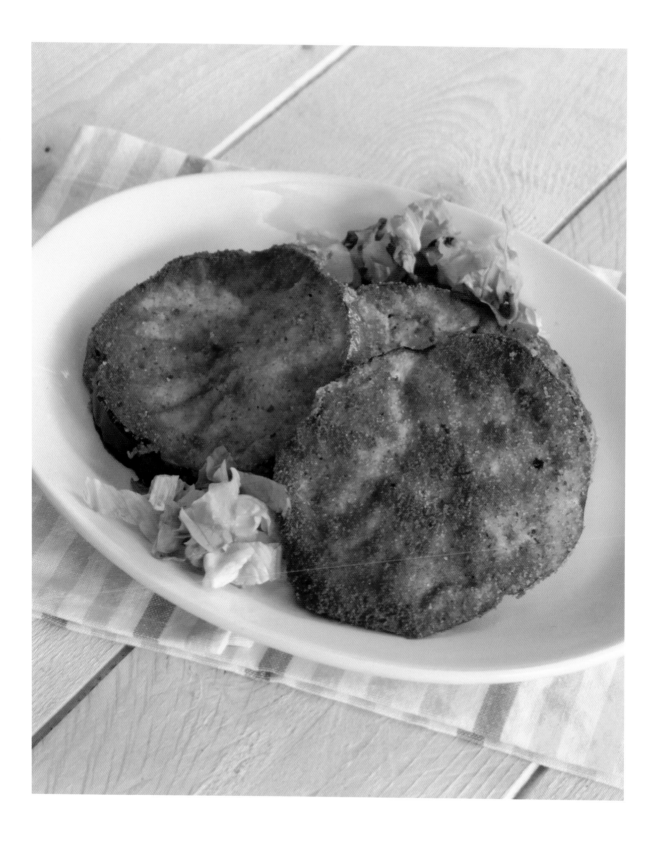

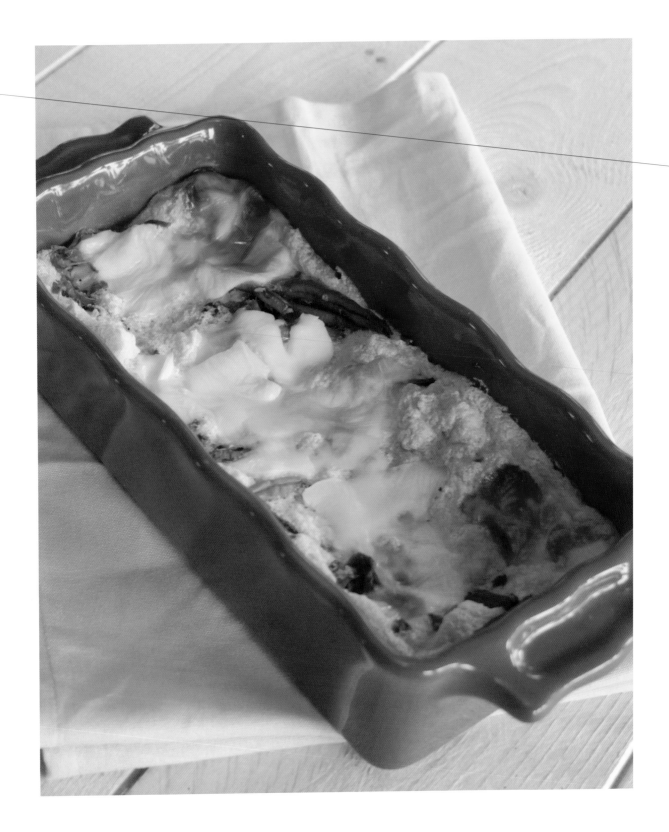

*In Italian, "Tortino" means a little cake, flourless, made with seasonal vegetables, eggs and cheeses.*
*This recipe is recommended in the spring when the beans are fresh.*
*Typical cheeses of the Italian tradition give personality to the recipe, ensuring a very special taste. You can replace the cheeses in the recipe with Fontina cheese or semi-mature cheeses.*

# GREEN BEAN AND PROVOLONE CAKE

## (TORTINO DI FAGIOLINI E PROVOLONE)

### VEG

### *Serves 2*

## INGREDIENTS

- 500 g (1 lb 2 oz) green beans, trimmed
- 2 eggs
- 200 ml (7 fl oz) milk
- 5 tablespoons grated Parmigiano cheese
- pinch of nutmeg
- 100 g (3½ oz) Asiago cheese, diced
- 150 g (5½ oz) Provolone cheese, diced
- extra virgin olive oil, to taste
- sea salt and pepper, to taste

## METHOD

Preheat the oven to 180°C (350°F/Gas 4). Lightly grease and line a 22 cm (8½ inch) springform tin with baking paper

Boil the green beans in salted water for 5 minutes. Drain.

Beat the egg yolks with the milk, Parmigiano and nutmeg.

Add the cheeses, oil, salt, pepper and mix well. Add the egg whites.

Pour a layer of green bean in the tin, Then add a layer of the egg mixture. Add another layer of green beans and then the egg mixture until you have used all of the ingredients.

Baked for 20–25 minutes. Serve warm or cold.

*A modern twist on Panzanella, a 'poor' dish (piatto povero) of the Tuscan tradition whose name derives from 'bread to soak'. High-quality ingredients are essential for the success of a dish that is not 'just' a salad but a feast of Italian flavours.*

*The original recipe calls for the use of the red onion, vinegar and bread soaked in water, then squeezed and crumbled. Over time, the recipe was modified with the addition of other ingredients such as tomatoes, olives and mozzarella.*

# PANZANELLA SALAD

(PANZANELLA)

V

*Serves 2*

## INGREDIENTS

- 15 cherry tomatoes, halved
- 2 small red onions, chopped
- 10 basil leaves, roughly chopped
- oregano, roughly chopped, to taste
- 2 slices of rustic bread, toasted and cut into cubes
- sea salt, to taste
- white pepper, to taste
- extra virgin olive oil, to taste

## METHOD

Place the vegetables in a bowl and add the basil and oregano. Gently toss. Add the bread.
Season with the salt, pepper, a generous amount of olive oil and stir.
Allow to stand for at least 30 minutes to allow the flavours to mix together.

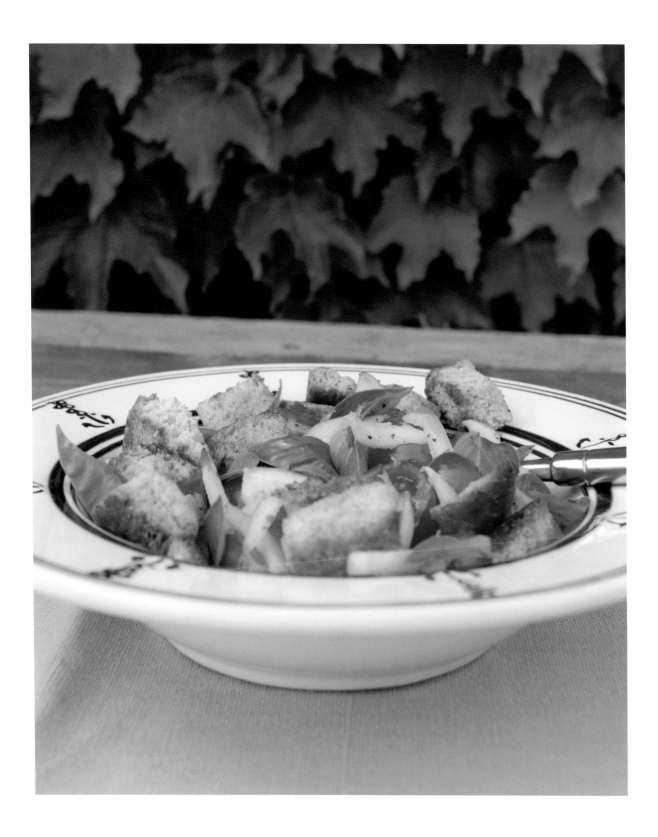

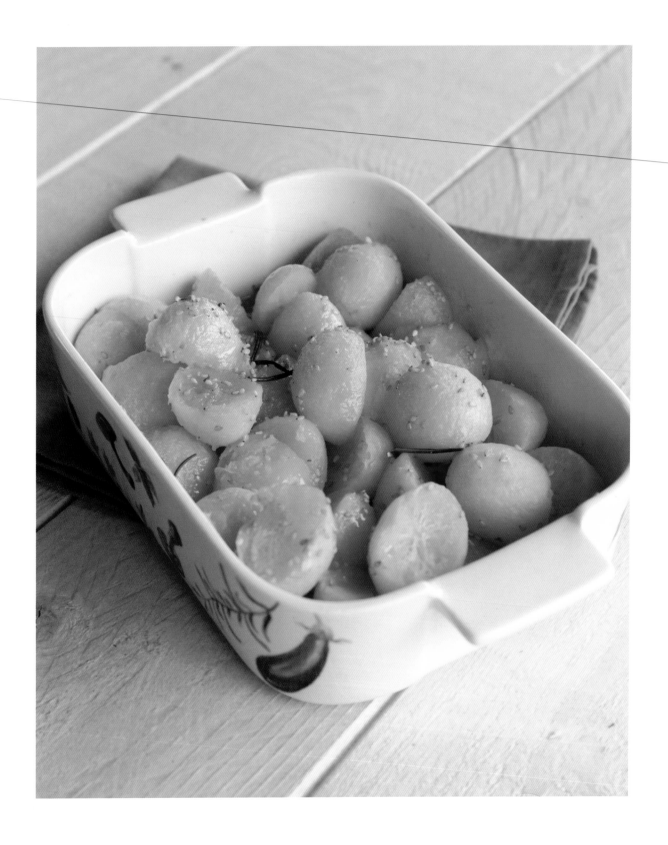

*Sesame seeds are a valuable source of nutrients. There are two types of sesame seeds: black and white. Their nutritional properties are very similar, even if the white sesame seeds are more easily available. The intake of sesame seeds is beneficial for bones, improves liver functions, stimulates circulation and helps to improve digestion. Beyond the benefits, the sesame seeds enrich a simple dish like this, with their scent and their crunchiness.*

# POTATOES WITH SESAME

(PATATE CON SESAMO)

EF-V

*Serves 4*

## INGREDIENTS

· 500 g (1 lb 2 oz) new potatoes
· 3 tablespoons white sesame seeds
· 1 teaspoon turmeric
· white pepper, to taste
· extra virgin oil, to taste
· sea salt, to taste

## METHOD

Cut in the potatoes half. Put the potatoes in a large pot and add enough water to cover them completely. Bring the potatoes to the boil. Reduce the temperature and cook over medium–low heat for about 15 minutes. When you can pierce them with a fork, they will be ready. Leave to cool and remove the peel (optional choice, especially if the potatoes are organic).

Preheat the oven to 180°C (350°F/Gas 4). Lightly grease a baking tin.

Add the potatoes to the tin with the sesame seeds, turmeric, pepper and salt. Toss gently to coat. Bake for 5–10 minutes. Serve hot.

*Radicchio is one of the most valuable Italian vegetables. From autumn to late winter, it colours the table with its unmistakable deep red. Radicchio is very versatile and elegant. Even a simple dish like this becomes delicious with the combination of a few select ingredients.*

# RADICCHIO WITH MASHED POTATOES

(RADICCHIO CON PUREA DI PATATE)

EF-VEG

*Serves 2*

## INGREDIENTS

- 5 potatoes
- pinch of sea salt
- pepper, to taste
- 1 tablespoon grated Parmigiano
- 250 ml (9 fl oz) milk (or rice milk)
- 1 onion
- 2 tablespoons extra virgin olive oil, to taste
- 1 tablespoon balsamic vinegar
- 1 tablespoon brown sugar
- 1 round radicchio
- 1 rosemary sprig

## METHOD

Steam the potatoes. Once cooked, drain and add the grated Parmigiano and milk and mash.

Heat 1 tablespoon of oil in a saucepan over medium heat. Add the onion and cook for about 10 minutes, adding water if necessary. Add the vinegar and brown sugar and continue cooking for a further 5 minutes.

Cut the radicchio into strips. Sauté for a few minutes with 1 tablespoon of oil. Remove from the heat, add the onion mixture and mix.

Pour the mashed potatoes into a serving dish, cover with vegetables and garnish with a sprig of rosemary, soaked in extra virgin olive oil.

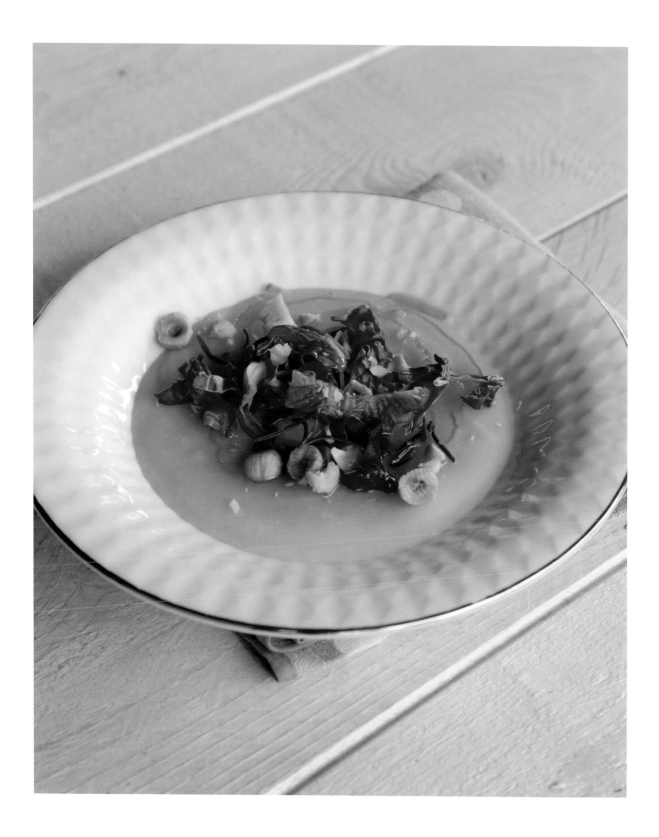

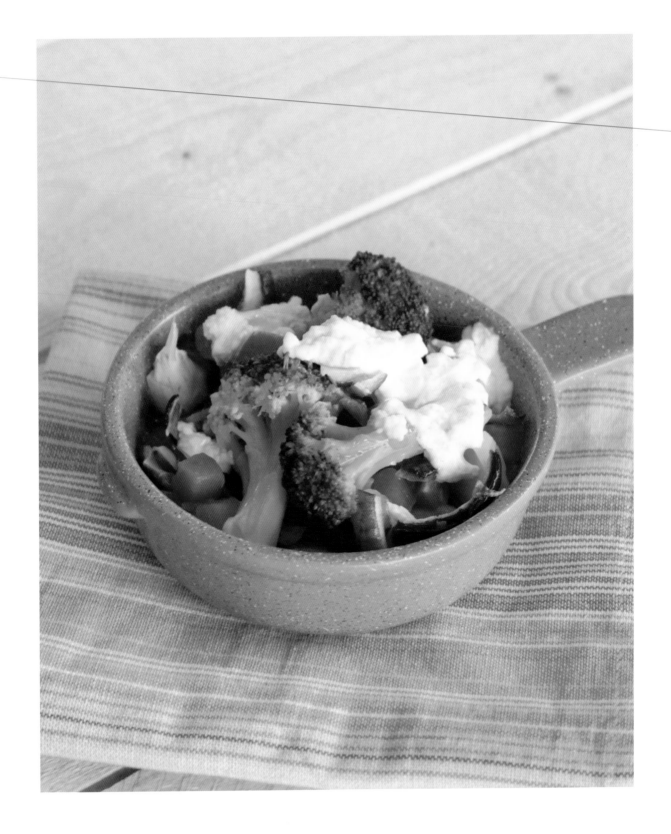

*A diet rich in vegetables is not only healthy but also fun because you can cook them in so many ways. This "timballo" is delicious and can be served in a cocotte portion, preferably freshly baked.*

# VEGETABLE PIE

## (TIMBALLO DI VERDURE)

EF-VEG

*Serves 4*

**INGREDIENTS**

- 200 g (7 oz) onion, chopped
- 400 g (14 oz) pumpkin (winter squash), chopped
- 400 g (14 oz) potatoes, chopped
- pinch of sea salt
- 400 g (14 oz) broccoli florets
- 100 g (3½ oz) soft cheese (or rice cheese for a vegan recipe), cut into cubes
- extra virgin olive oil, to taste

**METHOD**

Preheat the oven to 180°C (350°F/Gas 4). Lightly grease and line a baking tin with baking paper.

Place the onions, pumpkin and potatoes in a bowl and season with salt.

Boil the broccoli florets in boiling salted water for 5 minutes.

Arrange the vegetables in layers in the tin, alternating with the cheese. Cover with aluminium foil and bake for 25 minutes.

*The creamy zucchini (courgette) soup is also ideal cold. I love to add feta to it. This is one of those spring comfort foods that I can't give up. Italian parsley from my garden is my added extra.*

# ZUCCHINI SOUP

(CREMA DI ZUCCHINE)

GF-V

*Serves 2*

**INGREDIENTS**

- 4 zucchini (courgettes), sliced
- 1 onion, julienned
- 2 large potatoes, cut into cubes
- extra virgin olive oil, to taste
- pepper and sea salt, to taste
- 1 flat-leaf (Italian) parsley sprig
- 4 ladles water

**METHOD**

Heat 3 tablespoons of oil in a frying pan over medium heat. Add the onion and brown for about 10 minutes. Add the zucchini and potatoes and cook for 5 minutes.

Add 4 ladles water, bring to the boil and cook for 20 minutes, or until the vegetables tender.

Remove from the heat, add salt and pepper and blend until frothy. Garnish with parsley.

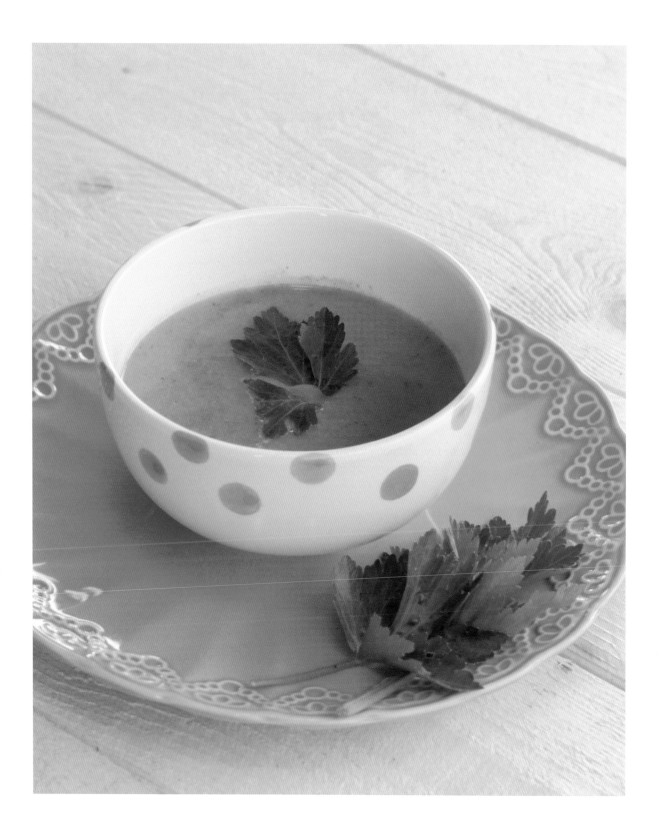

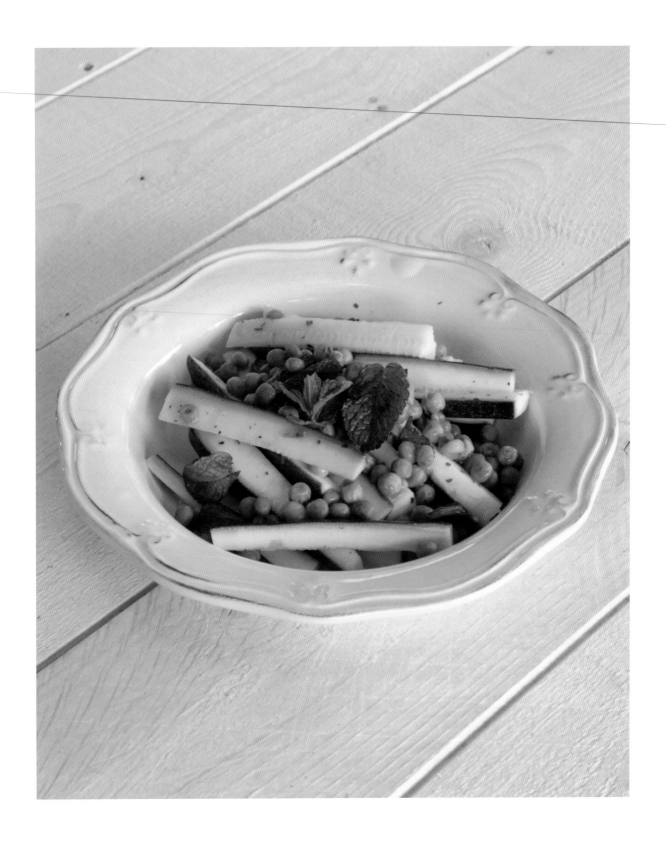

*A great side dish and when eaten with rustic bread, eggs or Parmigiano it also becomes a light main dish.*

# ZUCCHINI, PEAS AND MINT

(ZUCCHINE, PISELLINI E MENTA)

GF-V

*Serves 4*

## INGREDIENTS

- 1 lemon
- 5 zucchini (courgettes), cut into cubes
- extra virgin olive oil, to taste
- 6 mint leaves
- sea salt and pepper, to taste
- 200 g (7 oz) fresh peas

## METHOD

Wash the lemon, remove the zest and cut into strips.

Place the zucchini in a bowl. Add the oil, mint, salt and pepper and leave to marinate for 40 minutes.

Preheat the oven to 180°C (350°F/Gas 4). Lightly grease a baking tin.

Cook the peas in a saucepan of boiling salted water for 10–15 minutes.

Place the zucchini with the sauce in the baking tin, add the fresh peas and bake for 20 minutes. Serve hot.

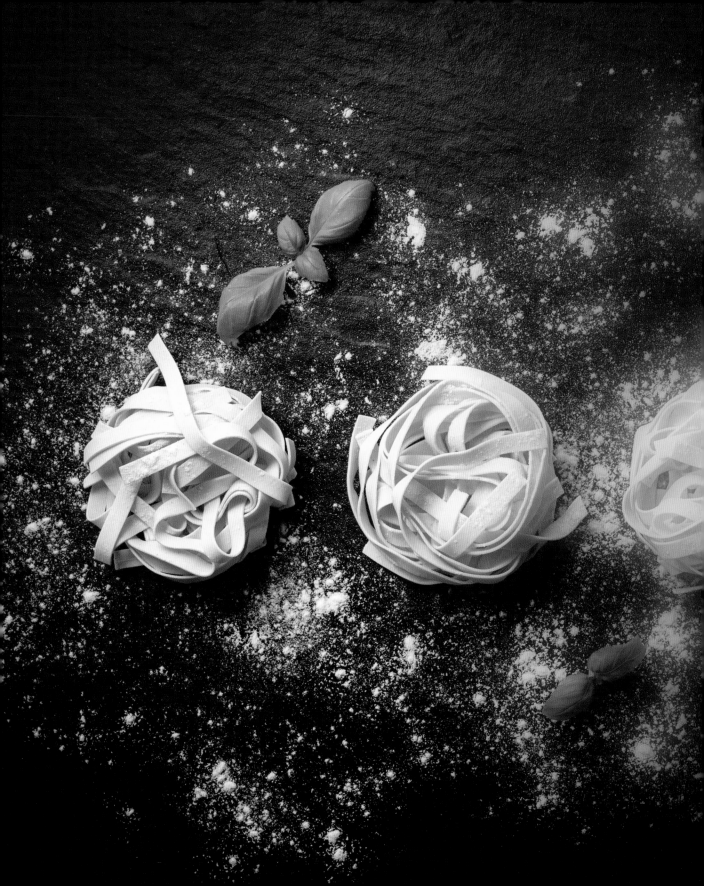

# PASTA & CEREALS

Pasta and cereals are the basics of Italian food, the cornerstones of the Mediterranean diet.

The Italian dried pasta, made with the durum wheat flour (or wholemeal flour of ancient Italian grain) is a daily food on the Italian table. In a short time and with simple, light seasonings, you can prepare a full and healthy dish.

The key is the quantity and the quality of the pasta (do not buy pasta made with soft flour. This is not real Italian pasta). The right daily amount of pasta never exceeds 80 g (2³/₄ oz). That's why Italians, while consuming pasta almost every day, do not get fat. Carbohydrates, consumed with vegetables, are essential to the body.

Grains such as rice, farro or the "fake" cereals such as buckwheat (it is a herbaceous plant) are equally present on Italian tables. Italy is one of the major rice producers. It is grown in Northern Italy where it is consumed, especially as "risotto". In the South, it is preferred in summer salads.

Wholegrains are an invaluable ally. Eaten *al dente*, they retain their nutritional properties and enhance the flavour of the seasonings. In some cases, they need cooking a little longer (which usually does not exceed 40 minutes) but it's worth it.

Simplicity is the basis of this recipe section. The natural cuisine needs just a few high-quality ingredients.

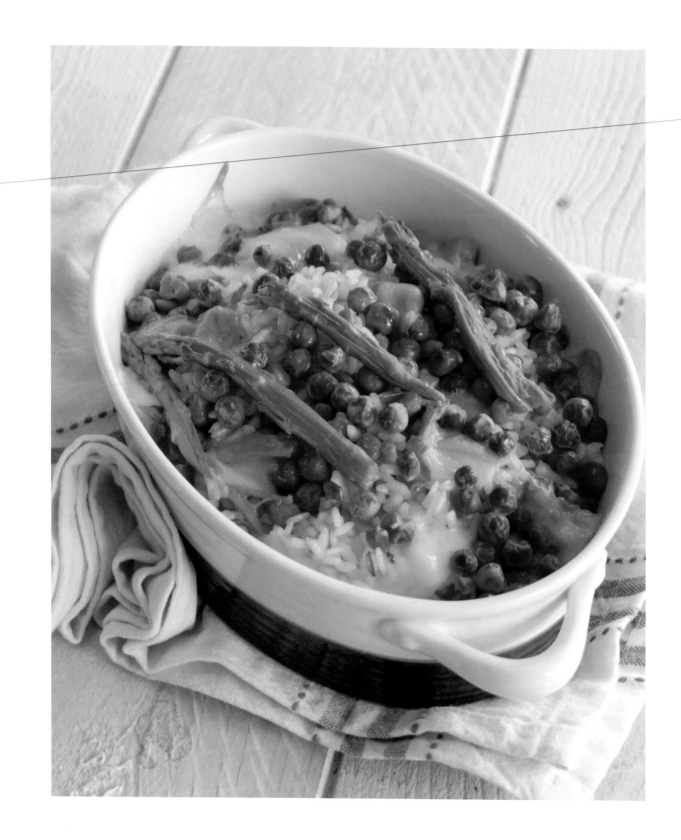

*I love baked rice. It is my favourite cooking method. I love the crispness of the surface and the soft interior texture, derived from vegetables and cheeses.*

*In spring, the pairing of asparagus and peas is one of my favourites. The onion adds a the special touch. The choice of cheese is not random. I find that the smoked Provola, with its characteristic taste, is perfect for this delicious dish.*

# BAKED BROWN RICE WITH PEAS AND ASPARAGUS

(RISO INTEGRALE AL FORNO CON PISELLI E ASPARAGI)

EF-GF-VEG

*Serves 4*

## INGREDIENTS

- 400 g (14 oz) brown rice
- 20 asparagus
- 150 g (5½ oz) fresh peas
- 1 spring onion (scallion), finely sliced
- extra virgin olive oil to taste
- 150 g (5½ oz) smoked Provola cheese, cut into cubes

## METHOD

Rinse the rice and drain. Cook the rice in a large saucepan of boiling salted water, following packet directions, until *al dente*. Drain and set aside until needed.

Clean the asparagus, removing the hardest part of the stem. Boil the asparagus in a saucepan of boiling salted water for about 10 minutes. Drain and set aside until needed.

Boil the peas in a saucepan of boiling salted water for 15–20 minutes (depending on their size. Fresh peas need a little longer to cook). Drain and set aside until needed.

Preheat the oven to 180°C (350°F/Gas 4). Grease a baking tin.

Heat some oil in a frying pan over medium heat. Add the onion and cook until brown. In the same pan, add the asparagus, peas and rice and mix to combine, adding 250 ml (9 fl oz) of water.

Pour the rice mixture into the baking tin and add the cheese on top. Bake for 20 minutes. Serve with extra cheese, if you like.

*The barley texture is ideal for this type of preparation and this recipe makes for a comforting lunch or dinner.*

# BARLEY SOUP WITH ROSEMARY

(ZUPPA DI ORZO AL ROSMARINO)

V

*Serves 2*

## INGREDIENTS

· 150 g (5½ oz) hulled barley
· 50 g (1¾ oz) green beans, trimmed
· 100 g (3½ oz) fresh peas
· 1 carrot, finely chopped
· 1 celery stalk, finely chopped

· 1 onion, finely chopped
· extra virgin olive oil, to taste
· pinch of sea salt
· pepper, to taste
· 1 rosemary sprig

## METHOD

Rinse the barley and drain. Cook the barley in a large saucepan of boiling salted water, following packet directions, until al dente. Drain and reserve 5 tablespoons of cooking water. Set aside until needed.

Cook the green beans in a large saucepan of boiling salted water for 10 minutes.

Cook the peas in a large saucepan of boiling salted water for 15–20 minutes.

Heat 1 tablespoon of oil in a frying pan over medium heat. Add the carrot, celery and onion and cook for 1–2 minutes. Add the green beans, peas and barley and stir. Add the reserved cooking water, some pepper and the chopped rosemary. Cook for 5 minutes, stirring occasionally. Serve hot.

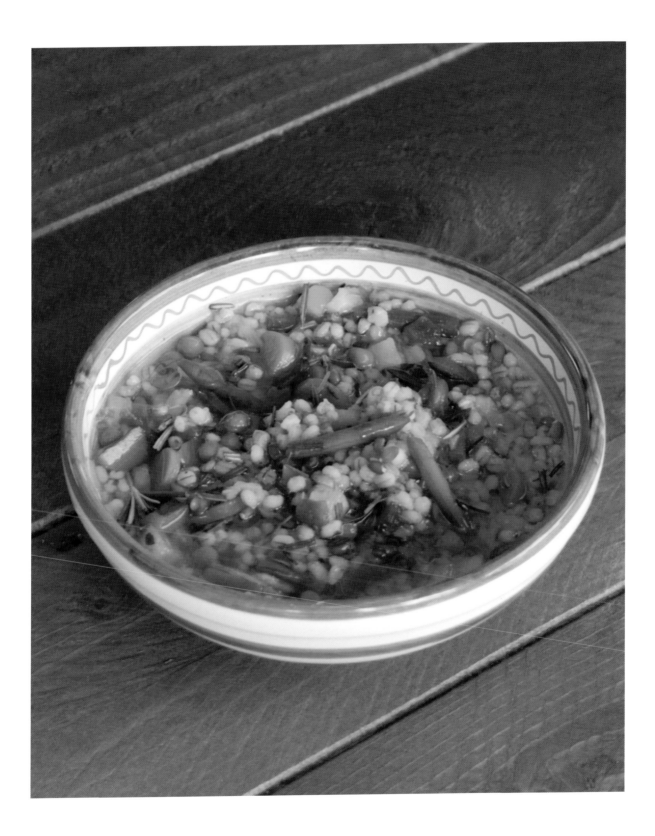

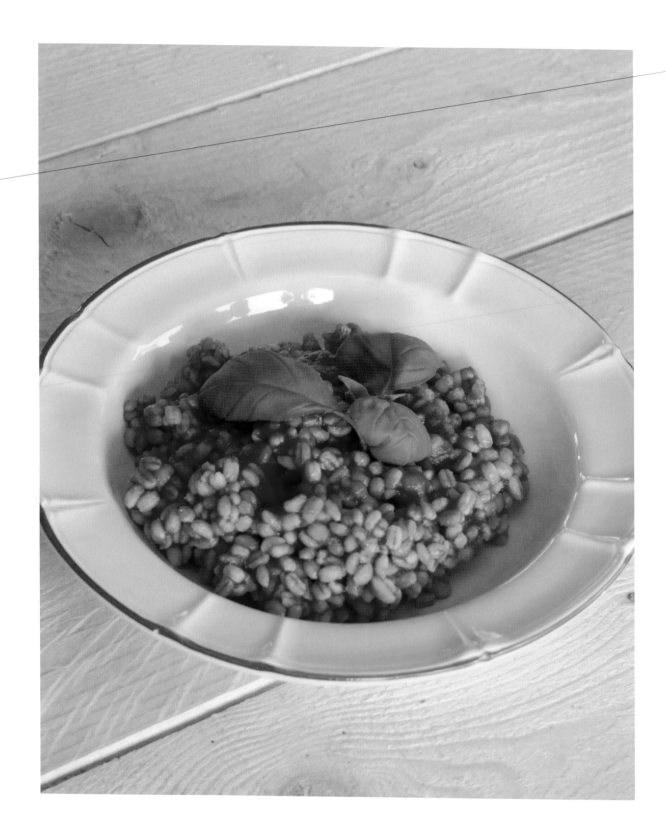

*Tomatoes and Parmigiano are two essential ingredients in a true Italian pantry. They give life to dishes with a unique flavor and there is no need to add more. Of course, you can replace barley with brown rice, even if I think barley, especially in spring and summer is an unbeatable, hearty combination.*

# BARLEY WITH TOMATO SAUCE AND PARMIGIANO

(ORZO CON POMODORO E PARMIGIANO)

EF-GF-VEG

*Serves 4*

## INGREDIENTS

· 400 g (14 oz) fresh tomatoes (for sauce)
· 1 garlic clove, finely chopped
· 1 onion, finely chopped
· 1 basil sprig
· 140 ml (4³/₄ fl oz) extra virgin olive oil
· 300 g (10¹/₂ oz) hulled barley
· 5 tablespoons grated Parmigiano

## METHOD

Blanch the tomatoes in a saucepan of boiling water for 1 minute. Remove the skin and seeds and chop.

Heat 3 tablespoons of oil in a frying pan over medium heat. Add the garlic and onion and fry gently for 2 minutes. Add the tomatoes, basil and cook for 15 minutes, adding salt during cooking.

Rinse the barley and drain. Cook the barley in a large saucepan of boiling salted water, following packet directions, until al dente. Drain and set aside until needed.

Add the barley to the sauce and mix. Add the Parmigiano and serve.

*Pesto, as usual, is a typical summer dressing but in winter you can also prepare a tasty sauce.*

*Broccoli are particularly suitable for the preparation of a delicious winter pesto. They have an ideal texture, a delicate but rich taste and a beautiful colour that makes this dish perfect.*

# BROWN RICE WITH BROCCOLI PESTO

(RISO INTEGRALE CON PESTO DI BROCCOLI)

EF-GF-VEG

*Serves 4*

## INGREDIENTS

- 320 g (11¼ oz) brown rice
- 300 g (10½ oz) broccoli florets
- 1 tablespoon pine nuts
- 1 tablespoon toasted hazelnut

- 50 g (1¾ oz) grated Parmigiano
- 3 sage leaves
- pinch of sea salt
- 4 tablespoons extra virgin olive oil

## METHOD

Rinse the rice and drain. Cook the rice in a large saucepan of boiling salted water for 30 minutes, or following packet directions, until al dente. Drain and set aside until needed.

Blanch the broccoli in a saucepan of boiling salted water for 10 minutes. Strain and pour into a bowl with cold water (to prevent loss of bright colour).

When cool, add the broccoli to a food processor with the remaining ingredients and blend until creamy.

Combine the rice with the pesto and serve.

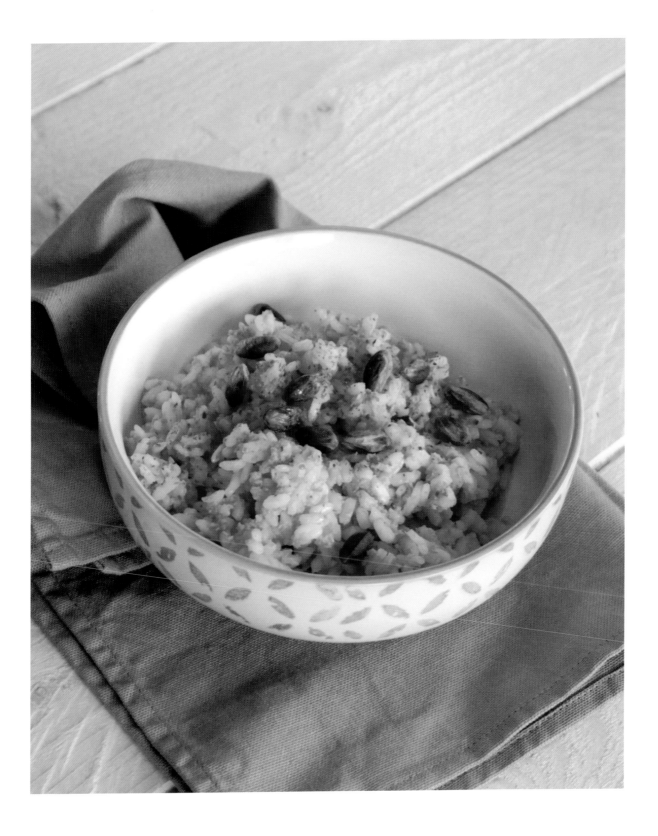

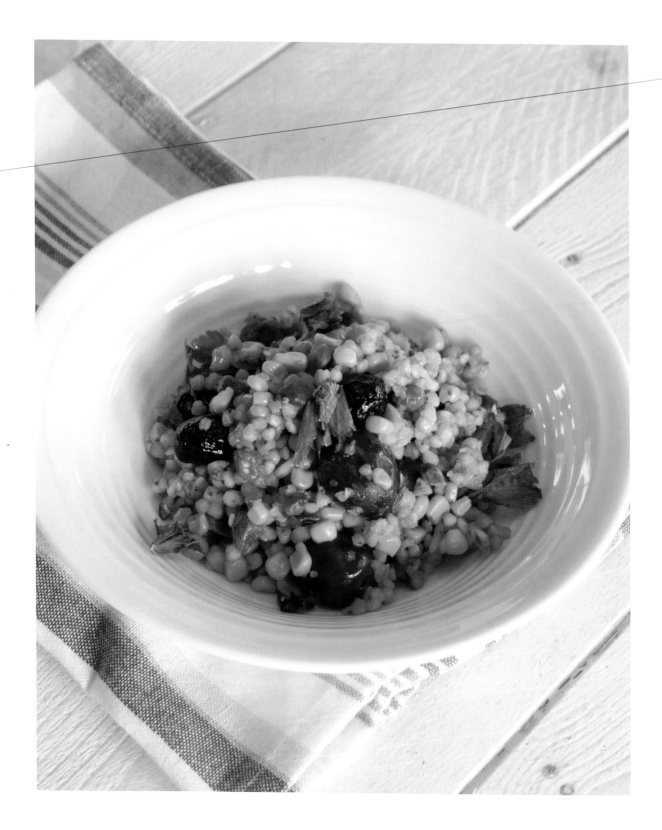

*Cereals are perfect in summer because they can be cooked the day before, dressed with oil and stored in the fridge to be served the next day. Rich in amino acids, buckwheat contains iron, zinc, selenium and potassium. It also contains certain antioxidants, including quercetin, which has anti-inflammatory properties and reduces blood pressure.*

*The key to this recipe is the corn kernels. They add sweetness to the strong taste of buckwheat.*

# BUCKWHEAT SALAD

(INSALATA DI GRANO SARACENO)

GF-V

*Serves 4*

## INGREDIENTS

- 250 g (9 oz) buckwheat
- juice of 1 lemon
- 100 ml (3½ fl oz) extra virgin olive oil
- 1 tablespoon finely chopped flat-leaf (Italian) parsley

- pinch of sea salt
- 1 celery stalk, sliced
- 1 tablespoon pitted black olives, sliced
- 1 tablespoon de-salted capers
- 3 tablespoons corn kernels

## METHOD

Rinse the buckwheat and drain. Cook the buckwheat in a large saucepan of boiling salted water for 15 minutes, or following packet directions. Drain and cool under running water. Set aside until needed.

In a bowl, emulsify the lemon juice, olive oil, parsley and salt. Add the citronette to the celery, olives, capers and corn and mix to combine.

Add the buckwheat to the vegetables and mix to combine. Leave to stand for 20 minutes before serving.

*Not all dried tomatoes are equal. Choose organic if possible. This allows you to always have on hand a healthy and tasty product—even when fresh tomatoes are not in season. This sauce is very simple but it is so rich and addictive.*

# BUCKWHEAT WITH CAPERS AND SUN-DRIED TOMATOES PESTO

(GRANO SARACENO CON PESTO DI CAPPERI E POMODORI SECCHI)

GF-V

*Serves 4*

## INGREDIENTS

· 320 g (11¼ oz) buckwheat
· 2 tablespoons salted capers, rinsed
· 20 sun-dried tomatoes
· 1 teaspoon dry oregano

· 50 g (1¾ oz) toasted hazelnuts
· extra virgin olive oil, to taste
· sea salt, to taste

## METHOD

Rinse the buckwheat and drain. Cook the buckwheat in a large saucepan of boiling salted water following packet directions. Drain and cool under running water. Set aside until needed.

Using a blender or food processor, blend the capers, tomatoes, oregano and hazelnuts, adding extra virgin olive oil to taste. Add sea salt to taste.

Combine the buckwheat with the sun-dried tomato mixture and serve.

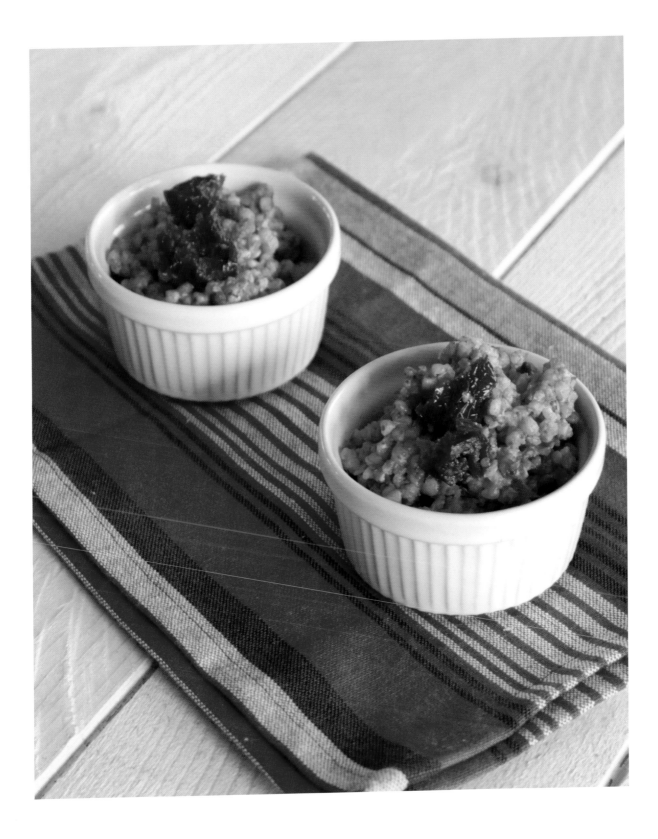

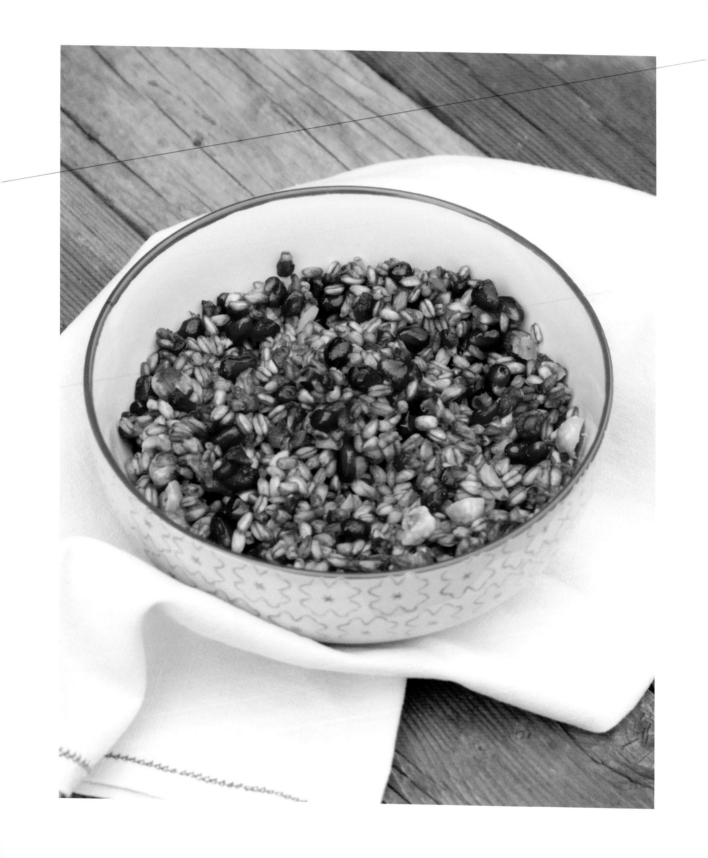

*This recipe is the perfect mix of beauty, health and taste. Rich in vitamin A and B, the pomegranate, according to Greek mythology, was a sacred plant and, to this day, it is a symbol of wealth and good fortune.*

*Farro is one of my favourite cereals. For the preparation of this salad you can choose wholegrain (whole-wheat) or pearl farro, remembering that cooking times will vary. Whole farro needs to soak for about 6 hours, while pearl does not need soaking. Cooking the farro, after soaking, takes between 45–60 minutes. This dish is perfect as main but it can also be served warm or cold as an appetizer in a single portion.*

# FARRO SALAD WITH WALNUTS AND POMEGRANATE

(INSALATA DI FARRO CON NOCI E MELAGRANA)

EF-DF-VEG

*Serves 2–4*

## INGREDIENTS

- 250 g (9 oz) pearl farro
- 4 tablespoons extra virgin olive oil
- 1 ripe pomegranate
- juice of 1 lemon
- 10 hazelnuts, roughly chopped
- pinch of white pepper
- pinch of sea salt

## METHOD

Rinse the farro and drain. Cook the farro in a large saucepan of boiling salted water, following packet directions, stirring occasionally, until *al dente*. Drain. Place the farro in a bowl, pour over the olive oil and set aside.

Remove the seeds from the pomegranate and squeeze the lemon juice over them.

Combine the remaining ingredients with the farro. Season with sea salt and white pepper and serve.

*Radicchio and burrata is a refined combination, rich in flavour and even nutritional properties. It is not always easy to find burrata but try Italian specialty stores.*

*Of course, this dressing goes well also with pasta, although the farro gives a special touch.*

# FARRO WITH RADICCHIO AND BURRATA

(FARRO CON RADICCHIO E BURRATA)

EF-VEG

*Serves 4*

## INGREDIENTS

- 320 g (11¼ oz) Farro (better if hulled)
- 1 head of radicchio, chopped
- 250 g (9 oz) PDO Burrata from Apulia, roughly chopped
- extra virgin olive oil, to taste
- pinch of sea salt
- pepper, to taste

## METHOD

Rinse the farro and drain. Cook the farro in a large saucepan of boiling salted water, following packet directions, until *al dente*. Drain, reserving 4–5 tablespoons of the cooking water. Set aside until needed.

Heat some oil in a frying pan over medium heat. Add the radicchio and salt and pepper and cook for 5 minutes. Add the reserved faro cooking water to the radicchio.

Add the Farro to the radicchio and mix. Add the burrata and remove from the heat, stirring to combine. Serve immediately.

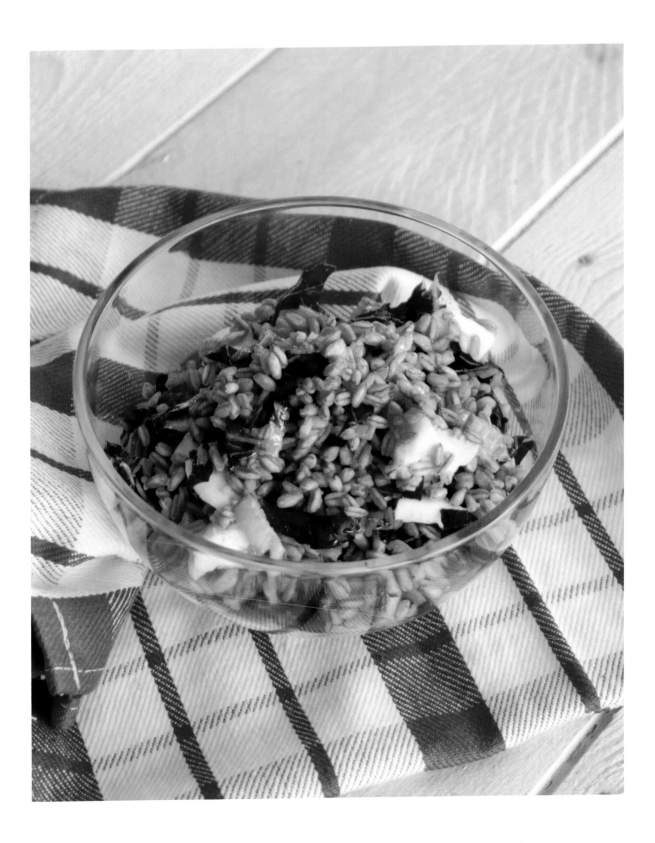

The so called 'poor dishes' of Italian culinary tradition, come from peasant traditions or, in some cases, from the kitchen during the time of the two World Wars. For many Italian families at this time, some foods were a real luxury. Meat was one of these foods, often replaced with legumes (defined as the 'poor man's meat'). Italians gave life to dishes that today are considered true 'cult' meals, such as pasta with fake sauce. Originating in Sicily, this dish roughly follows the same method for ragu sauce but without meat, and this is where the name 'fake sauce' comes from. Light and with a very special taste, this sauce is perfect with the first tomatoes of late spring.

# WHOLEMEAL PASTA WITH FAKE SAUCE

(PASTA INTEGRALE AL SUGO FINTO)

V

*Serves 4*

## INGREDIENTS

· 1 garlic clove, finely chopped
· 1 onion, finely chopped
· extra virgin olive oil, to taste
· 1 tablespoon red wine
· 1 carrot, finely chopped

· 300 g (10$^1$/$_2$ oz) cherry or date tomatoes, chopped
· 100 g (3$^1$/$_2$ oz) sun-dried tomatoes in oil, chopped
· 6 basil leaves
· sea salt, to taste
· 320 g (11 oz) (wholemeal) whole-wheat short pasta

## METHOD

Heat a few tablespoons of olive oil in a frying pan over low heat. Add the garlic and onion and brown. Add the red wine and let it evaporate.

Add the cherry tomatoes and carrot to the pan. Cook for 15 minutes. Add the sun-dried tomatoes and season with salt.

Remove the sauce from the heat and add the basil leaves.

Cook the pasta in a large saucepan of boiling salted water, following packet directions, until *al dente*. Drain.

Combine the pasta with the fake sauce and serve

*I love artichokes and, as soon as their season starts, I eat them almost every day.*

*This dish is also perfect served warm. For a more natural taste, it is preferable to use fresh artichokes hearts and not the ones packed in oil.*

# FUSILLI WITH ARTICHOKES

(FUSILLI CON CARCIOFI)

EF-VEG

## Serves 4

### INGREDIENTS
- 8 artichoke hearts
- 1 red onion, finely chopped
- 200 g (7 oz) smoked Provola cheese, cut into cubes
- extra virgin olive oil, to taste
- 1 glass white wine
- 320 g (11¹/₄ oz) wholemeal (whole-wheat) fusilli, or other short pasta
- pinch of sea salt
- white pepper, to taste

### METHOD
Divide the artichoke hearts in half and cut into thin slices.

Heat some oil in a saucepan over medium heat. Add the onion and fry for 1–2 minutes, then add the artichokes and cook for 2 minutes. Add the white wine, let it evaporate, cover and cook for 10 minutes.

Cook the pasta in a large saucepan of boiling salted water, following packet directions, until al dente. Drain and set aside until needed.

Combine the pasta with the artichokes. Add the cheese and pepper. Serve with a splash of olive oil.

*Sicily and southern Italy are places full of lemons and it is easy to see why they are used in many dishes.*
*Usually for this recipe I use lemons from my garden. Choose organic lemons as it is critical to make the most of all the taste of the essential oils contained in the peel.*

# MEZZE PENNE WITH LEMON

(MEZZE PENNE AL LIMONE)

EF-V

*Serves 4*

## INGREDIENTS

· 1 lemon
· 50 g (1³/₄ oz) sliced almonds
· 5 tablespoons extra virgin olive oil
· 2 garlic clove, crushed
· 320 g (11¹/₄ oz) mezze penne, or other short pasta
· 80 g (2³/₄ oz) Pecorino cheese, grated
· 5 mint leaves

## METHOD

Wash the lemon, grate the zest and squeeze the juice.

Toast the almonds in a dry frying pan over medium heat.

Heat the oil in a frying pan over medium heat. Add the garlic and brown.

Cook the pasta in a large saucepan of boiling salted water, following packet directions, until al dente. Drain, reserving some of the cooking water, and set aside until needed.

Add the pasta to the pan with the oil and garlic and mix. Remove the garlic. Add the lemon juice. Sprinkle with pecorino, and add some of the reserved cooking water. Serve with lemon zest, almonds and mint.

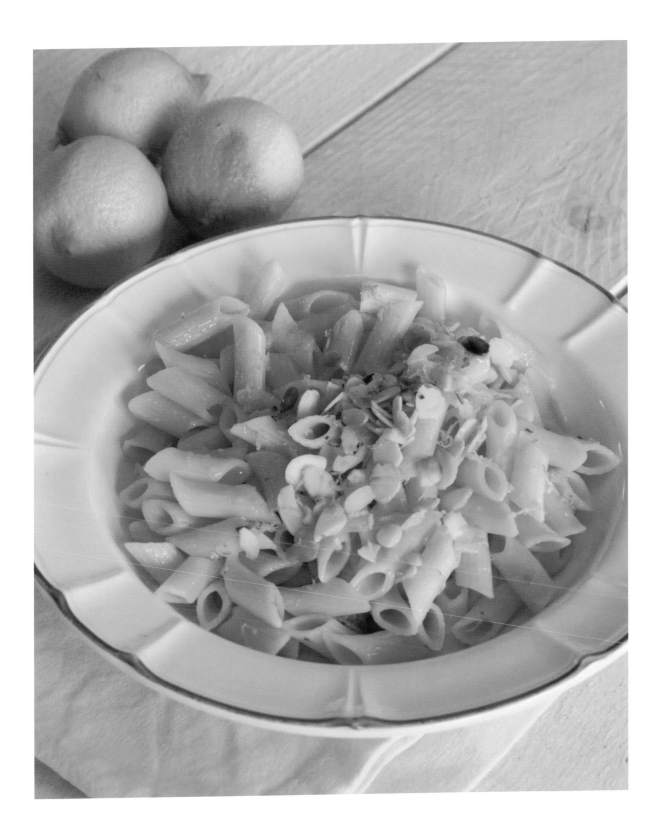

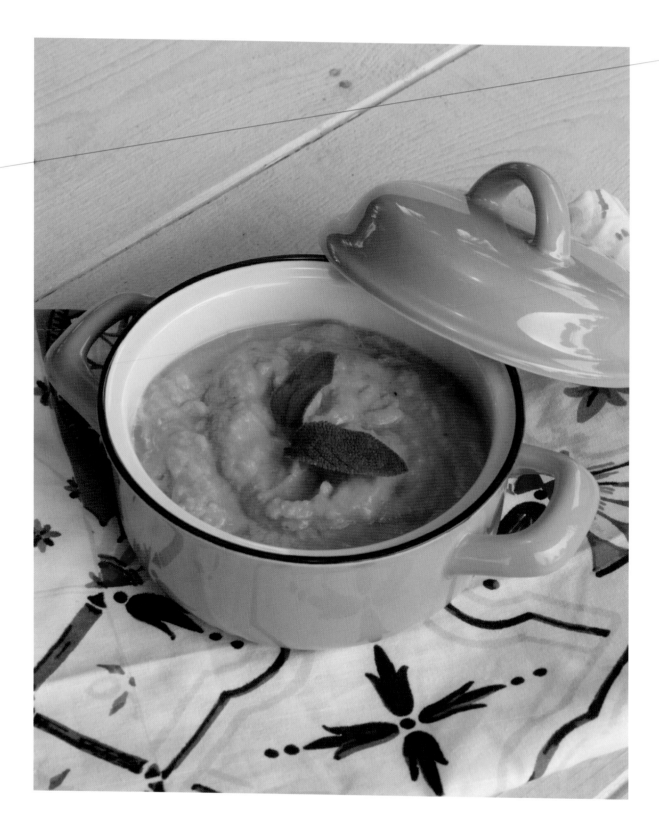

*Combining cereals with legumes is ideal from a nutritional point of view. A perfect comfort food in the cold months.*

*You can replace the chickpeas with beans or lentils, although I find the combination of oats and chickpeas irresistible.*

# OAT AND CHICKPEA SOUP

(ZUPPA DI AVENA E CECI)

V

*Serves 4*

## INGREDIENTS

- 200 g (7 oz) oats
- 200 g (7 oz) chickpeas
- 2 carrots, finely diced
- 1 celery stalk, finely chopped
- 1 onion, finely sliced
- 1 tablespoon rosemary
- pinch of sea salt
- 2 potatoes, cut into cubes
- extra virgin olive oil, to taste

## METHOD

In two separate bowls, soak the oats and chickpeas in cold water overnight (add a pinch of baking soda to beans, this will make them softer).

The next day, drain the chickpeas and oats and cook in a large pot over medium heat. Add the carrots, celery, onion, rosemary and salt and cook over low heat for 50 minutes, covering with a lid. Halfway through cooking, add the potatoes. Add the salt.

Remove from the heat, add the extra virgin olive oil and serve hot.

*A typical dish of southern Italy, Orecchiette is a variety of pasta from the Puglia (Apulia) region. It is available both fresh and dry, made with durum wheat semolina and is great when eaten with seasonal broccoli. Pecorino enhances this simple but very tasty dish, which is always present on the winter Italian table.*

# ORECCHIETTE WITH BROCCOLI AND PECORINO

(ORECCHIETTE CON BROCCOLI E PECORINO)

VEG

*Serves 4*

## INGREDIENTS

- 500 g (1 lb 2 oz) broccoli
- 1 onion, finely chopped
- extra virgin olive oil, to taste
- pinch of sea salt
- Pepper, to taste
- 320 g (11¼ oz) dry or fresh orecchiette pasta
- Grated pecorino cheese, to taste

## METHOD

Cut the broccoli, eliminating the hardest parts and steam.

Heat some oil in a frying pan over medium heat. Add the onion and brown. Add the broccoli florets and salt and pepper and cook, stirring for 2–3 minutes.

Cook the pasta in a large saucepan of boiling salted water, following packet directions, until *al dente*. Drain and set aside until needed.

Combine the pasta and broccoli. Add the Pecorino and serve immediately.

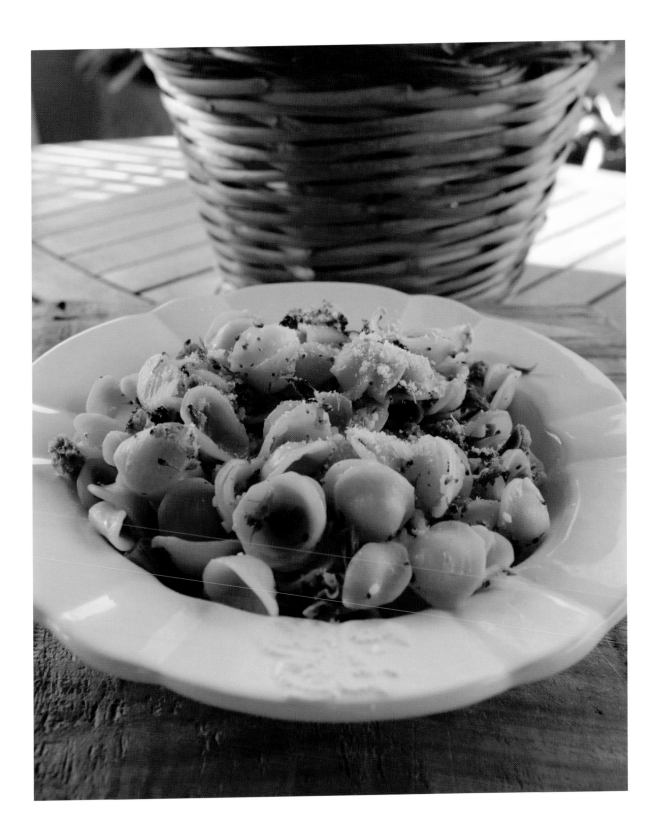

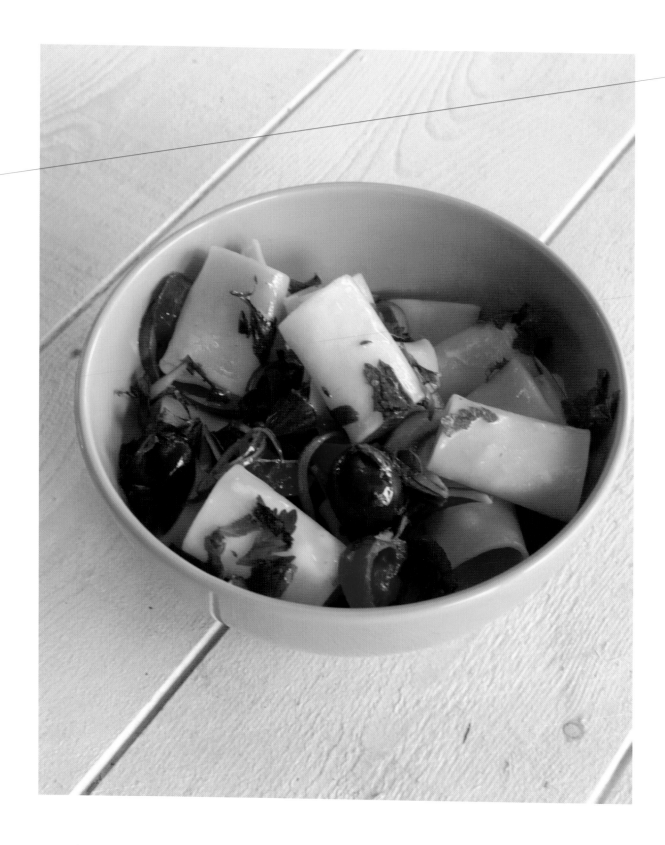

*This is a classic of summer Italian cuisine. A fresh and light dish. In addition, it is also a perfect dish on the go. Just make the salad a few hours before, or the night before.*

*The key to this recipe is al dente pasta which is highly digestible.*

# PASTA SALAD

(INSALATA DI PASTA)

V

*Serves 4*

## INGREDIENTS

- 1 red onion, finely sliced
- 5 tomatoes, finely diced
- 1 parsley sprig
- 1 tablespoon pitted olives
- extra virgin olive , to taste
- pinch of sea salt
- 300 g (10½ oz) short pasta

## METHOD

Soak the onion in cold water for 20 minutes. Drain.

Combine the tomatoes, onions, parsley and olives in a bowl and season with olive oil and salt.

Cook the pasta in a large saucepan of boiling salted water, following packet directions, until *al dente*. Drain and set aside until needed.

Add the pasta to salad and mix to combine. Leave to stand for about 20 minutes before serving.

*Asparagus and Caprino (goat cheese) are a delicious combination. The pungent flavor of the asparagus is damped by the delicacy of this mild Italian cheese I love very much.*

# PASTA WITH ASPARAGUS AND CAPRINO CHEESE

(PASTA CON ASPARAGI E CAPRINO)

EF-VEG

*Serves 2*

## INGREDIENTS

- 250 g (9 oz) asparagus
- 100 g (3½ oz) green beans, trimmed
- 1 spring onion (scallion)
- 300 g (10½ oz) wholemeal (whole-wheat) short pasta
- 200 g (7 oz) Caprino (goat) cheese (or ricotta)
- 50 g (1¾ oz) grated Parmigiano cheese

## METHOD

Clean the asparagus, removing the final part. Boil in a saucepan of boiling salted water for about 10–15 minutes (depending on thickness).

Cook the green beans in a saucepan of boiling salted water until *al dente*.

Heat some oil in a frying pan over medium heat. Add the onion and brown. Add the asparagus and green beans and mix to combine.

Cook the pasta in a large saucepan of boiling salted water, following packet directions, until *al dente*. Drain, reserving 2 tablespoons of the cooking water.

In a bowl, mix the soft cheese with the reserved cooking water.

Add the pasta to the vegetables, then add the cream and mix. Serve hot or warm with grated Parmigiano.

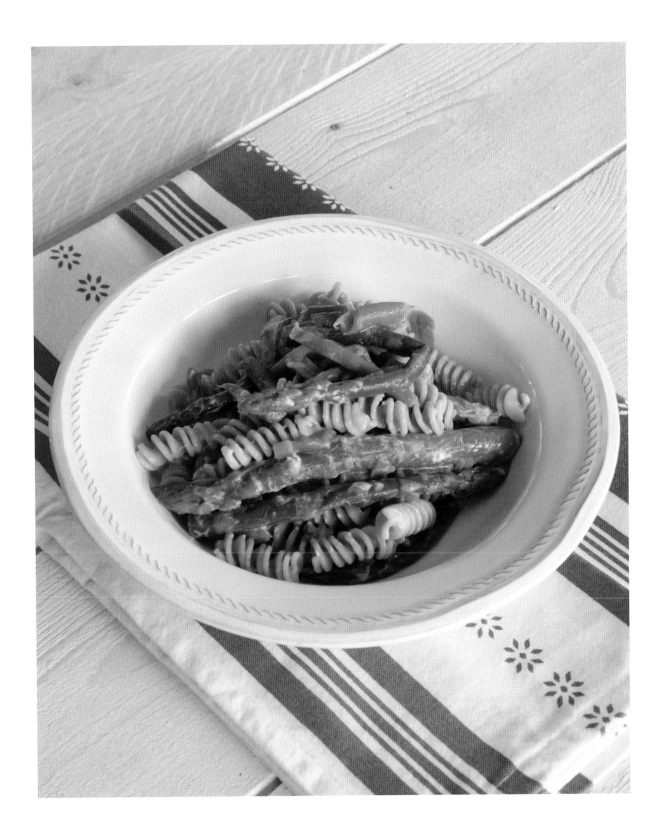

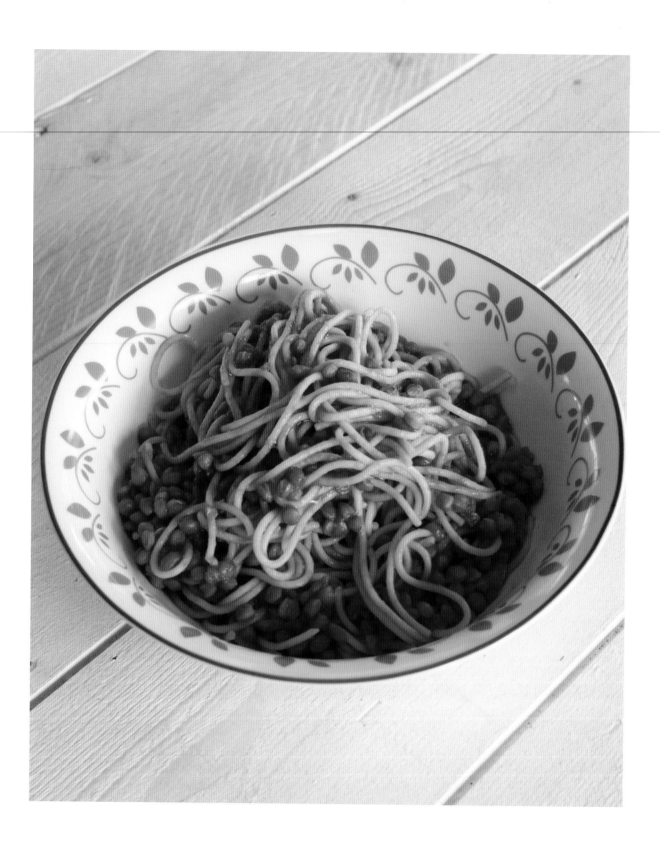

*This is a complete meal that combines the complex carbohydrates of pasta with the natural proteins of lentils. The tomato sauce is the key to a sauce that can be considered a true delicious Italian vegan ragu.*

# PASTA WITH LENTILS SAUCE

(PASTA CON RAGU DI LENTICCHIE)

V

*Serves 4*

## INGREDIENTS

· 2 carrots, finely chopped
· 1 celery stalk, finely chopped
· 1 onion, finely chopped
· 250 g (9 oz) lentils, rinsed
· 250 ml (9 fl oz) tomato pasta sauce
· 500 ml (17 fl oz) warm water

· 300 g (10½ oz) pasta (long or short, to your liking)
· extra virgin olive oil, to taste
· pinch of sea salt
· pepper, to taste

## METHOD

Heat the oil in a thick-bottomed pan. Add the carrot, celery and onion and stir. Cover with a lid and cook until the vegetables are soft.

Add the lentils to the vegetables. Add the tomato sauce and cover with hot water.

Bring to the boil, reduce the heat to low and leave to simmer for 30 minutes, stirring occasionally. Towards the end of cooking, add salt and pepper.

Cook the pasta in a large saucepan of boiling salted water, following packet directions, until *al dente*. Drain.

Add the pasta to the pan with the lentils. Mix well and serve still warm.

*This is a true winter comfort food and a hearty meal. Walnuts, hazelnuts and tomatoes are a delicious combination. A full dish rich in taste you have to serve strictly hot.*

# PASTA WITH WALNUT AND HAZELNUT SAUCE

(PASTA CON SALSA DI NOCI E NOCCIOLE)

V

*Serves 4*

## INGREDIENTS

- 150 g (5½ oz) walnuts
- 50 g (1¾ oz) toasted hazelnuts
- 2 tablespoons tomato sauce
- 300 g (10½ oz) wholemeal (whole-wheat) short pasta

- rice milk, to taste
- extra virgin olive oil, to taste
- pinch of sea salt
- 1 flat-leaf (Italian) parsley sprig, chopped

## METHOD

Using a blender or food processor, mix the walnuts, hazelnuts, tomato sauce and rice milk, little by little until you get a cream.

Cook the pasta in a large saucepan of boiling salted water, following packet directions, until *al dente*. Drain.

Add the pasta to a pot over low heat and mix with the walnut sauce.

Garnish with the parsley and serve immediately.

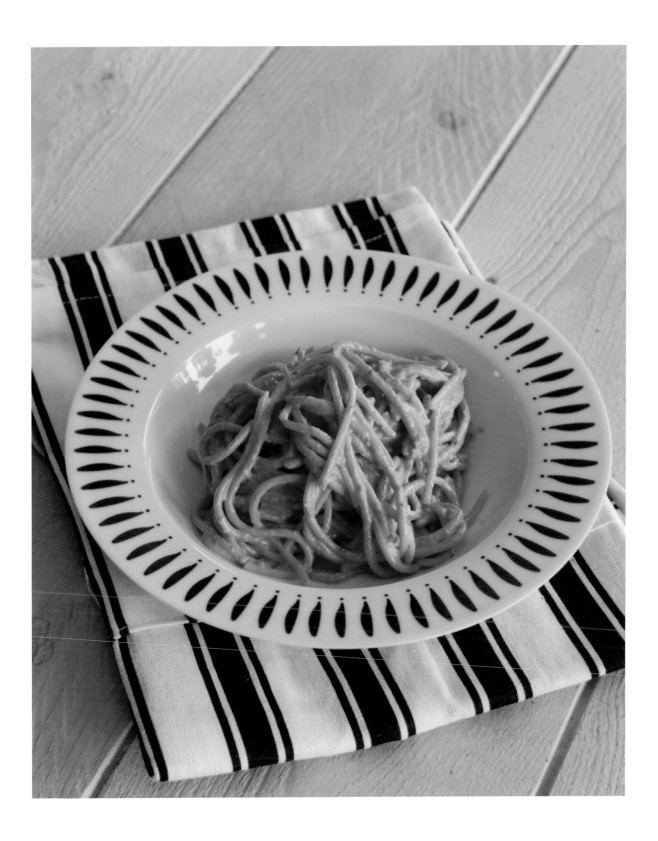

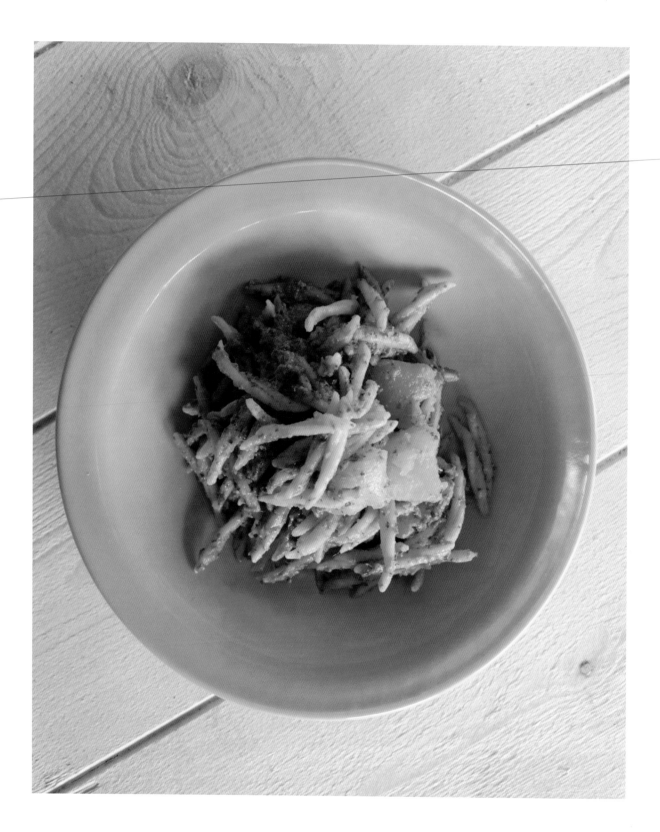

*This dish is a tribute to Liguria (northern Italy), a region full of culinary treasures. Trofie pasta and pesto are two of Liguria best-known symbols in the world.*

*When I was a child, my mother made this dish with potatoes. Even now, I find it's one of her winning dishes.*

# TROFIE PASTA WITH PESTO AND POTATOES

(TROFIE CON PESTO E PATATE)

EF-VEG

### *Serves 4*

**INGREDIENTS**

- 1 large bunch basil
- 1 garlic clove
- 50 g (1³/₄ oz) pine nuts
- 2 tablespoons grated Parmigiano

- 2 tablespoons Pecorino
- extra virgin olive oil, to taste
- 200 g (7 oz) potatoes, cut into cubes
- 300 g (10¹/₂ oz) trofie pasta (or other short pasta)

**METHOD**

Using a blender or food processor, blend the basil with the garlic, pine nuts, Parmigiano and Pecorino. Add olive oil.

Cook the potatoes in a large saucepan of boiling salted water for 5 minutes. Add the pasta and cook for 10–15 minutes.

Drain the pasta and potatoes, season with pesto and serve.

*The lightness of the ricotta and the delicate flavour of zucchini make this dish simply delicious.*

*Usually, Italians love to buy ricotta cheese from local producers who guarantee quality and convenience. These are two essential factors when it comes to food, especially for fresh cheese like ricotta.*

# SPAGHETTI WITH RICOTTA AND ZUCCHINI (COURGETTES)

(SPAGHETTI CON RICOTTA E ZUCCHINE)

EF-VEG

*Serves 4*

## INGREDIENTS

- 6 zucchini (courgettes), sliced
- 1 garlic clove
- 4 mint leaves, chopped
- pinch of sea salt
- extra virgin olive oil, to taste
- 300 g (10½ oz) ricotta
- 2 tablespoons milk
- 3 tablespoons grated Parmigiano
- 300 g (10½ oz) wholemeal (whole-wheat) spaghetti
- white pepper, to taste

## METHOD

Grill the zucchini on a barbecue chargrill plate or in a chargrill pan.

Place the zucchini in a bowl, add the garlic, mint leaves and a pinch of salt. Set aside.

Cook the pasta in a large saucepan of boiling salted water, following packet directions, until *al dente*. Drain.

Combine the ricotta with the milk and Parmigiano.

Combine the pasta, zucchini and ricotta cream and add a sprinkling of pepper. Serve.

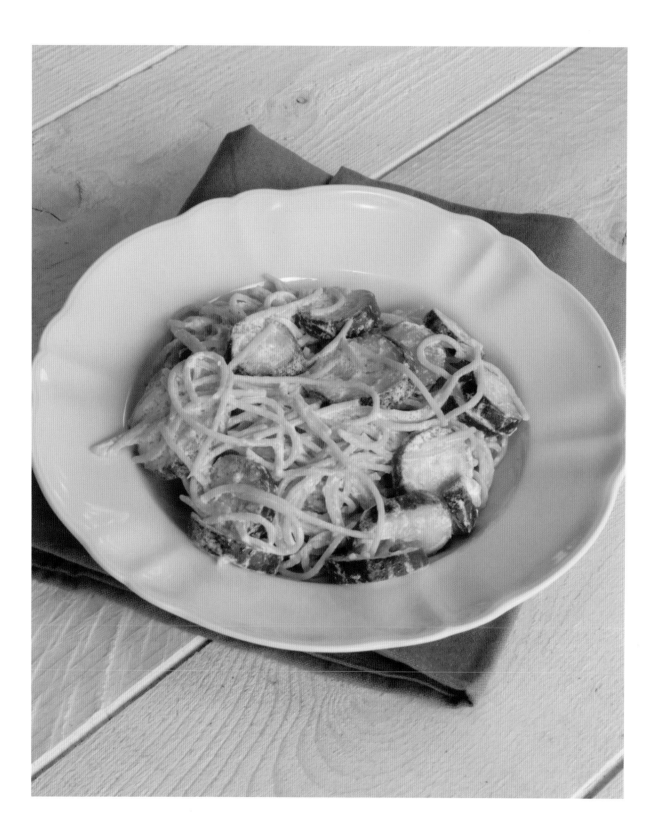

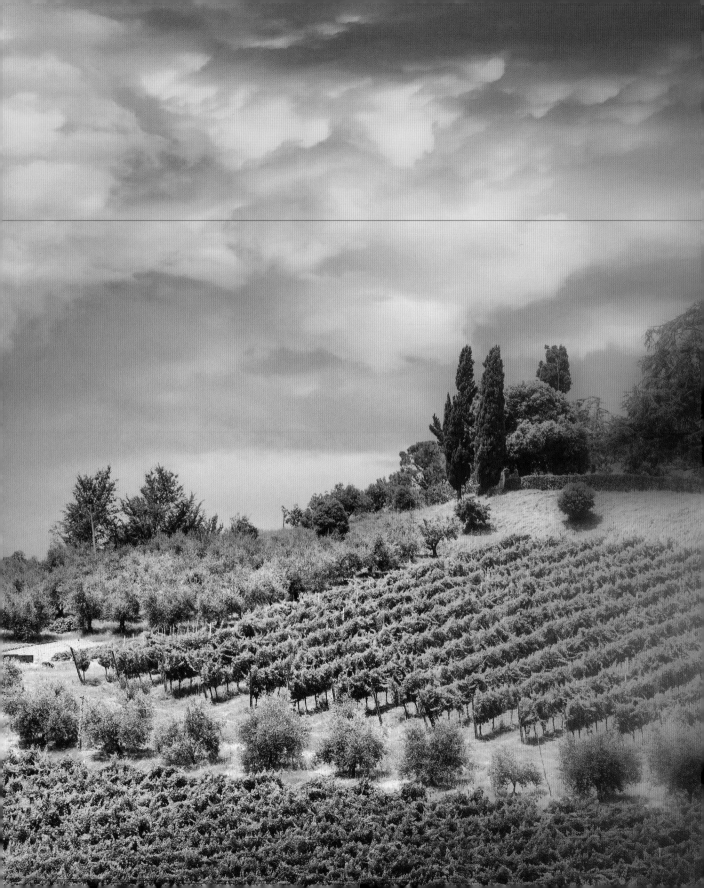

# VEGETARIAN AND VEGAN PROTEINS

In the Mediterranean diet, legumes are considered a valuable food. They have an excellent quality-price ratio, are available everywhere and all year long, and have a very high protein value. Once considered the 'meat of the poor', today legumes are noble foods, whose daily consumption is beneficial.

Even eggs are a precious food if you select organic and free range.

Tofu and Seitan are the best-known plant proteins of Asian cuisine. You can prepare delicious meals in no time and with little cooking.

This chapter offers luscious meat alternatives for those who love sustainable cuisine for people and the planet.

We have many opportunities to eat healthy and tasty food with protein alternatives. In this chapter, you will find simple recipes, so tasty and light enough to be eaten every day.

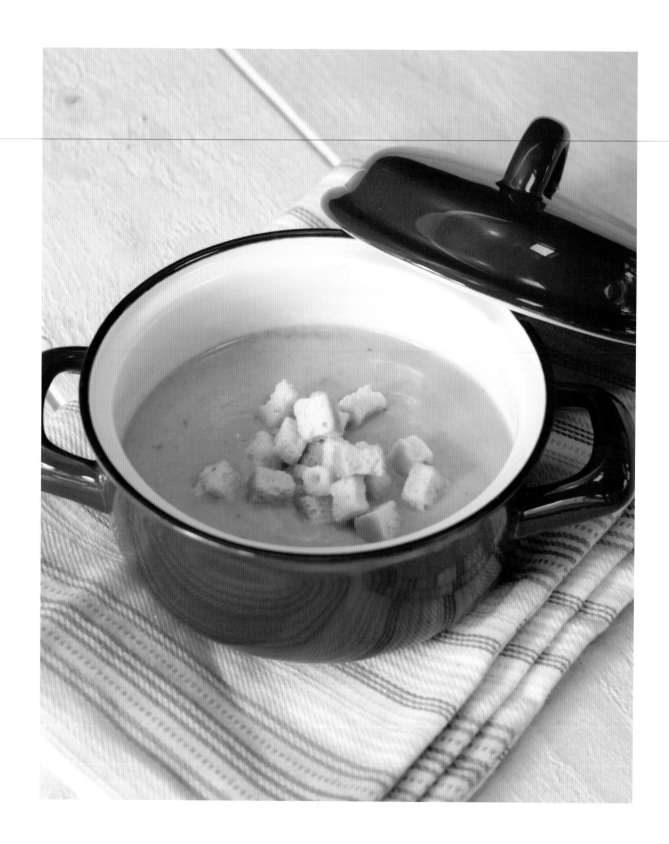

*There is a good amount of vegetable protein in this soup and, when accompanied by a second source of protein, like seitan (or tofu) it helps round out the meal.*

*Soups are a healthy meal if the vegetables are fresh. Soups are perfect to start a lunch and even more suitable for a light but nutritious dinner.*

# ARTICHOCKE AND CREAMY POTATO SOUP

(CREMA DI CARCIOFI E PATATE)

GF-V

*Serves 2-4*

## INGREDIENTS

· 300 g (10¹/₂ oz) potatoes
· 7 artichokes hearts
· 2 lemons, halved
· 1 celery stalk, finely chopped
· 1 carrot, finely chopped
· 1 onion, finely chopped
· 50 g (1³/₄ oz) pistachios

· 50 g (1³/₄ oz) walnuts
· 50 g (1³/₄ oz) whole almonds
· 2 slices of country style bread, roughly chopped
· extra virgin olive oil, to taste
· 300 ml (11 fl oz) warm water
· pinch of sea salt
· white pepper, to taste

## METHOD

Steam the potatoes. Aloow to cool, then peel and roughly chop.

Steam the artichoke hearts with the lemons.

Heat some oil in a frying pan over medium heat and add the celery, carrot and onion. Cook until browned.

Using a blender or food processor, process the potatoes, artichokes, chopped vegetables, pistachios, walnuts and almonds.

Add the bread, olive oil, warm water, salt and pepper and blend until desired consistency is reached (if necessary, add water).

Serve with a drizzle of olive oil and slices of toasted bread.

*A super-fast recipe which contains all the necessary nutrients and proteins.*
*Fresh vegetables and dried fruits are precious to those who choose a plant-based diet.*
*Brown rice should be eaten every day for its beneficial properties.*

# BROWN RICE WITH SPINACH AND TOASTED ALMONDS

(RISO INTEGRALE CON SPINACI E MANDORLE TOSTATE)

GF-V

*Serves 4*

### INGREDIENTS

· 320 g (11¼ oz) brown rice
· 400 g (14 oz) baby English spinach
· sea salt, to taste
· 1 garlic clove
· extra virgin olive oil, to taste
· 2 tablespoons chopped toasted almonds

### METHOD

Rinse the rice and drain. Cook the rice in a large saucepan of boiling salted water, following packet directions, until *al dente*. Drain and set aside until needed.

Heat some olive oil in a frying pan over medium heat. Add the spinach, salt and garlic and cook for a few minutes.

Add the rice and cook for 10 minutes, stirring. Serve hot with chopped toasted almonds.

*When cooked, Italian cannellini beans are delicious because of their soft texture and slightly nutty flavor. Available all year round, in winter, organic dried cannellini beans are the better choice while in summer, canned cannellini are perfect as they are ready to use. Rich in protein and vitamins, they are one of the bases of the Mediterranean diet.*

*This recipe is very easy to prepare and can be ready in a few minutes, with ingredients available in your garden or pantry. A good extra virgin olive oil is the key to this healthy salad.*

# CANNELLINI AND PACHINO TOMATO SALAD

(INSALATA DI CANNELLINI E POMODORI PACHINO)

V - GF

*Serves 4*

## INGREDIENTS

· 12 cherry tomatoes, halved
· 1 onion, sliced
· extra virgin olive oil, to taste
· sea salt and white pepper, to taste

· dried oregano, to taste
· 300 g (10¹/₂ oz) canned cannellini beans, rinsed and drained.

## METHOD

Combine the tomatoes and onion and season with olive oil, salt, pepper and oregano. Set aside for about 10 minutes.

Add the beans to the tomato mixture, toss gently to combine and serve.

*If the presence of pear seems odd, the result will surprise you. A hearty dish with a very refined taste.*

# CHICKPEA AND PEAR CREAMY SOUP

(CREMA DI CECI E PERE)

GF-V

*Serves 4*

## INGREDIENTS

- 1 onion, finely diced
- 1 celery stalk, finely sliced
- extra virgin olive oil, to taste
- 2 carrots, finely diced
- 1 teaspoon paprika
- 1 pear, finely diced
- 200 g (7 oz) cooked chickpeas
- 500 ml (17 fl oz) warm water
- pinch of sea salt

## METHOD

Heat some oil in a frying pan over medium heat. Add the onion and celery and brown the onion for a few minutes.

Add the carrots to the pan with the paprika. Cover with hot water and bring to the boil.

After 10 minutes, add the chickpeas and pear. Cook until the carrots are soft enough. Add a pinch of sea salt.

Using a blender, blend the soup until creamy. Serve hot.

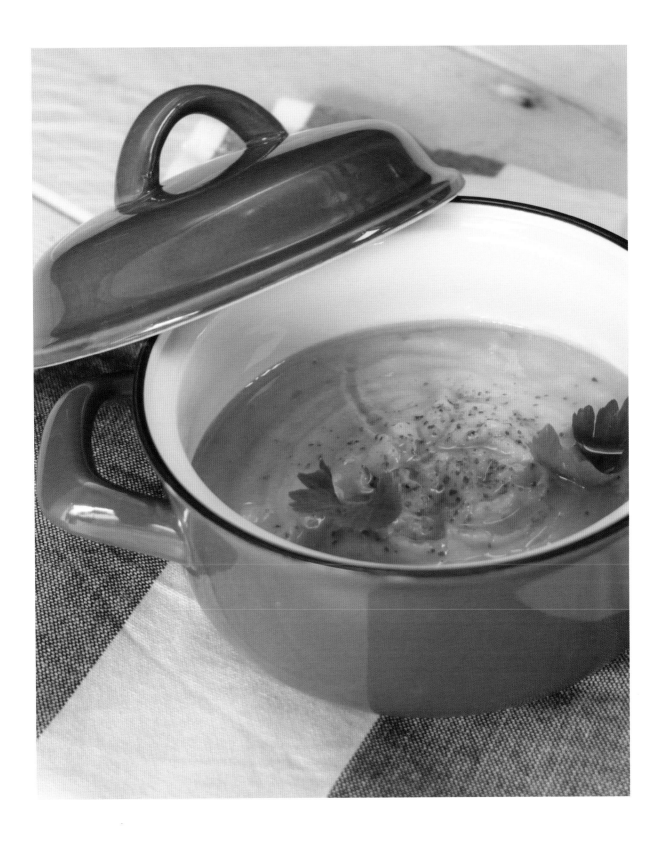

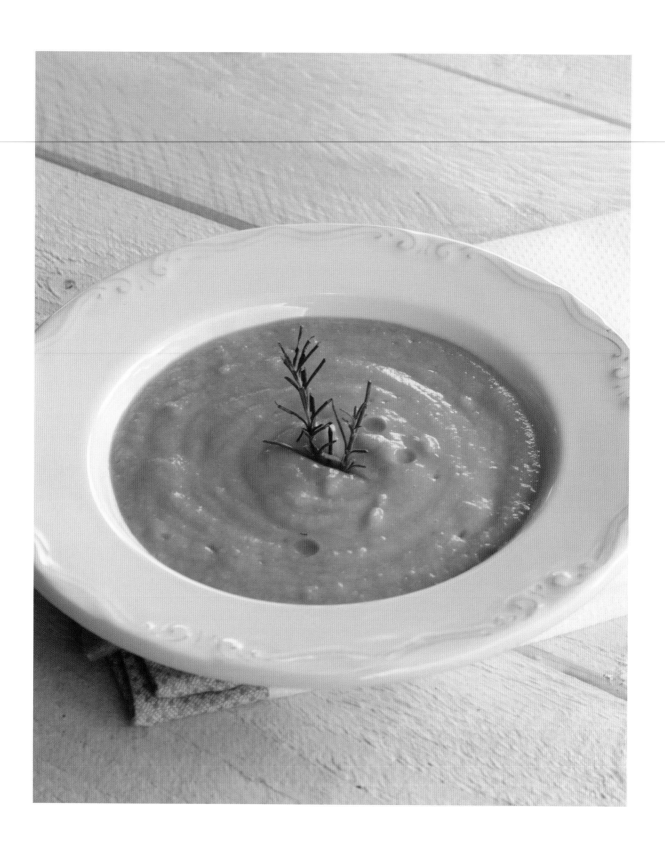

*Chickpeas and pumpkin are the perfect match for a soup with a velvety texture.*
*Rosemary emits a scent that is the key to this soup.*

# CHICKPEA AND PUMPKIN CREAMY SOUP

(VELLUTATA DI CECI E ZUCCA)

GF-V

*Serves 2*

## INGREDIENTS

- 250 g (9 oz) chickpeas
- 400 g (14 oz) pumpkin (winter squash) flesh, cut into cubes
- 1 onion, sliced into rings
- 1 tablespoon tomato pasta sauce
- 500 ml (17 fl oz) vegetable broth
- extra virgin olive oil, to taste
- pinch of sea salt
- pepper, to taste
- 1 rosemary sprig

## METHOD

Soak the chickpeas with a pinch of baking soda overnight. The next day, drain the beans and cook for 50 minues, adding salt at the end of cooking.

Place the pumpkin and onion in a saucepan with 3 tablespoons of olive oil and a pinch of salt. Simmer for 10 minutes.

Add chickpeas and tomato pasta sauce and mix. Add the vegetable broth and cook for 5 minutes. Remove from the heat and allow to cool slightly.

Using a blender, blend the mixture until smooth.

Heat the soup over medium heat and serve hot with chopped rosemary.

*This is one of my favourite salads, one of those dishes that I prepare in the morning and take away when I'm dining out.*

*Although there are excellent restaurants where you can eat tasty plant-based dishes, all we can prepare with our hands is invaluable.*

# FARRO SALAD WITH ROCKET PESTO AND BOILED EGGS

(INSALATA DI FARRO CON PESTO DI RUCOLA E UOVA SODE)

VEG

*Serves 4*

## INGREDIENTS

- 300 g (10½ oz) hulled farro
- 100 g (3½ oz) rocket (arugula) pesto
- 5 basil leaves
- 1 tablespoon dried oregano
- pinch of sea salt
- 6 sun-dried tomatoes, plus extra 4–6 for garnishing
- extra virgin olive oil, to taste
- juice of 1 lemon
- 4 hard-boiled eggs, halved

## METHOD

Cook the farro in a saucepan of boiling salted water for 35 minutes.

Wash the rocket and basil and blend with the dried oregano, sun-dried tomatoes, olive oil and lemon juice until you get the desired consistency.

Pour the farro in a salad bowl and add the sun-dried tomatoes, hard-boiled eggs and pesto. Season with a generous amount of extra virgin olive oil. Serve immediately.

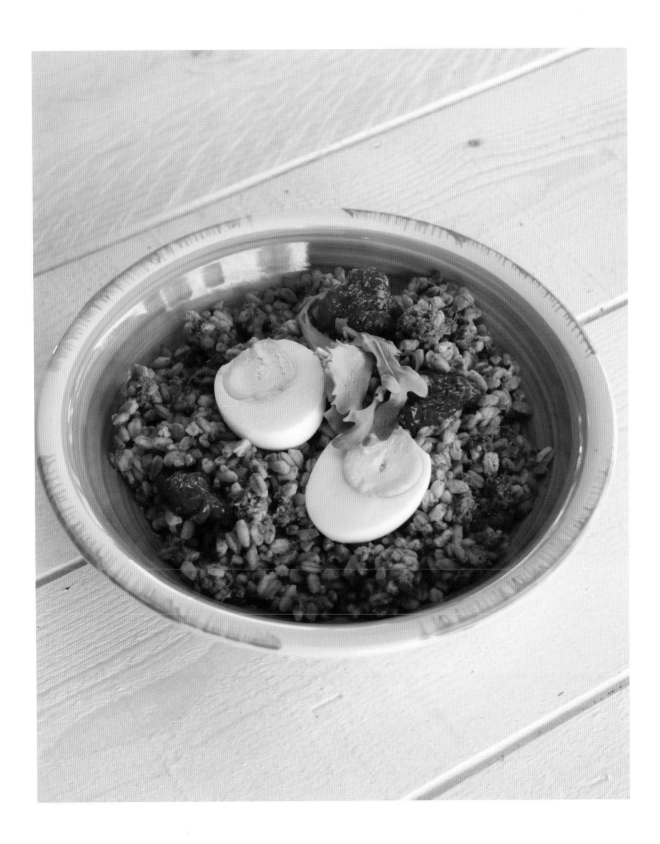

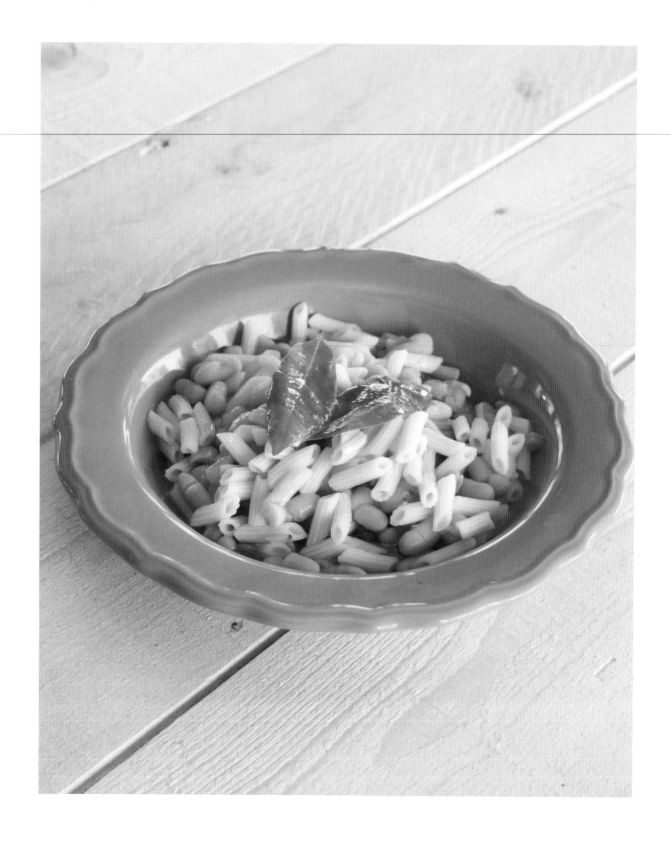

*In Italy, Minestrina (Literally 'little soup') is one of the best comfort foods. It is an invigorating dish to fight the flu and one of the dishes with which our grandmothers and mothers declare their love for their family.*

*Like many Italian recipes, there is not a traditional recipe because in every family there is a notebook in which the cook has added their favorite ingredient. Cannellini beans are my twist for this recipe.*

# HEARTY ITALIAN MINESTRINA

(MINESTRINA)

EF-VEG

*Serves 4*

## INGREDIENTS

- 300 g (10½ oz) dried cannellini beans
- 1 carrot, finely chopped
- 1 onion, finely chopped
- 1 celery stalk, finely chopped
- sea salt and pepper, to taste
- 1 bay leaf
- 320 g (11¼ oz) ditalini or stelline pastina
- extra virgin olive oil, to taste
- Parmigiano flakes

## METHOD

Soak the beans in cold water the night before.

Rinse and drain the beans. Add the beans to a saucepan with the carrot, onion and celery and cook for 1 hour.

Add the bay leaf and pasta and cook according to the packet directions.

Serve hot, with a generous helping of Parmigiano flakes.

*Polenta is a traditional dish in Northern Italian cooking that pairs deliciously well with meat alternatives such as lentils.*

*This recipe is easy and so delicious—perfect as winter comfort food.*

# LENTILS WITH POLENTA

(LENTICCHIE CON POLENTA)

GF-V

*Serves 4*

## INGREDIENTS

- 500 ml (17 fl oz) water
- 250 g (9 oz) pre-cooked polenta
- 1 celery stalk, finely chopped
- 1 carrot, finely chopped
- 1 onion, finely chopped
- 1 leek, finely chopped
- extra virgin olive oil, to taste

- pinch of sea salt
- 200 g (7 oz) lentils
- 250 ml (9 fl oz) white wine
- 400 g (14 oz) peeled tomatoes
- 1 teaspoon dried oregano
- pinch of sea salt
- pepper, to taste

## METHOD

Cook the polenta according the package directions. Set aside until needed.

Heat the oil in a large saucepan over medium heat. Add the vegetables with a pinch of salt. Cook gently for 15 minutes until everything is softened.

Stir in the lentils and deglaze with white wine. As soon as the wine has evaporated, add the tomatoes, oregano, salt and water and cook the lentils for 40 minutes, or until the lentils are tender. Add more water if needed.

Serve warm with hot polenta and a sprinkle of extra virgin olive oil.

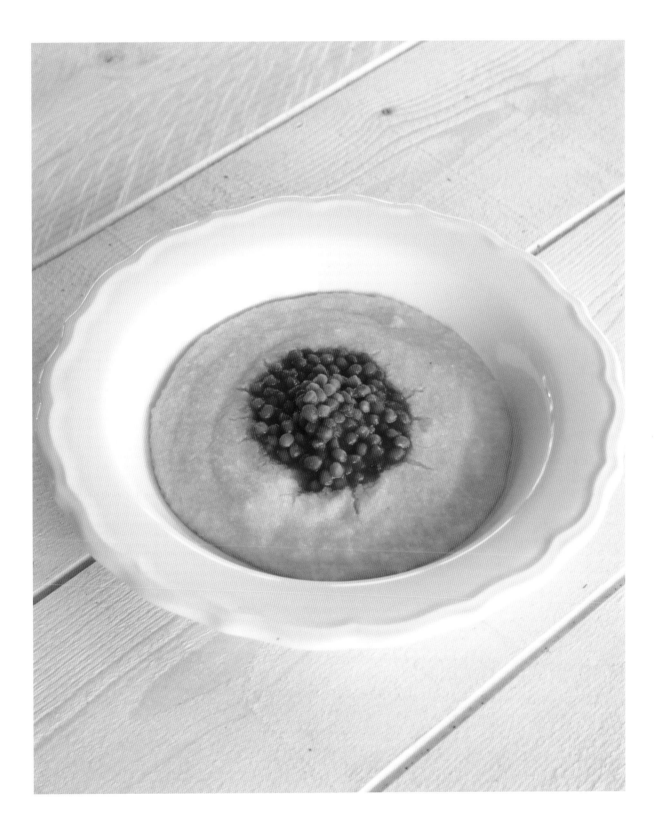

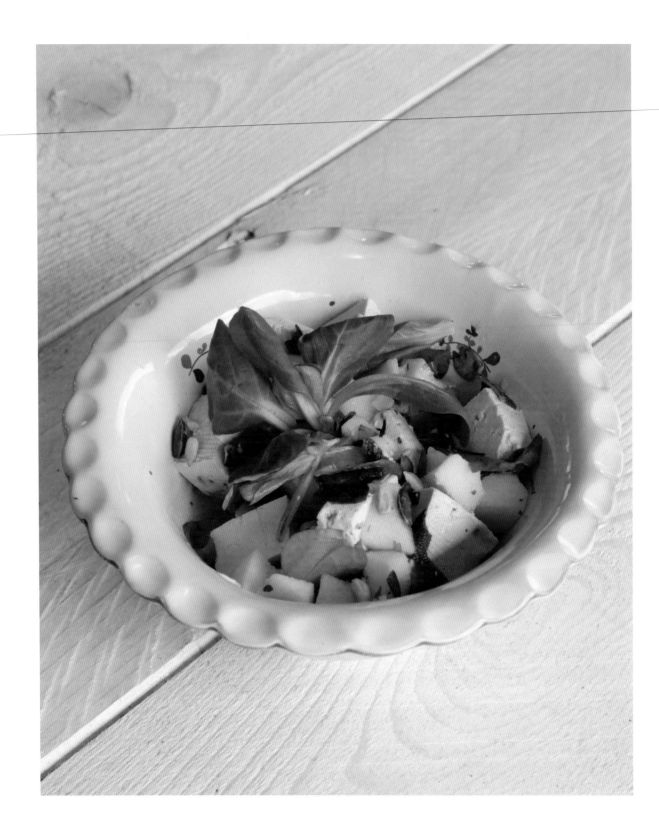

*Perfect as a summer dish, I love this recipe for its simple but firm taste.*
*The sesame and pumpkin seeds are the key ingredients to this fragrant recipe.*

# MARINATED TOFU

(TOFU MARINATO)

GF-V

*Serves 4*

**INGREDIENTS**

- 200 g (7 oz) natural tofu
- 1 lemon juice
- extra virgin olive oil, to taste
- sea salt, to taste
- pepper, to taste
- 1 tablespoon dried oregano
- 2 mint leaves
- 1 apple, finely diced
- 5 handfuls rocket (arugula)
- 2 tablespoons sesame seeds
- 2 tablespoons pumpkin seeds (pepitas)

**METHOD**

Dry and press the tofu in paper towels to squeeze out excess liquid. Cut into cubes.

Add the tofu to a bowl, add the lemon juice, oil, salt, pepper, oregano and mint leaves. Stir, then cover with a lid and refrigerate for 1 hour, stirring occasionally.

Pour the tofu in a serving dish. Sprinkle the apple with lemon juice and add to the bowl. Add the rocket, sesame seeds and pumpkin seeds. Serve.

*The red lentils are my favourite. They are much lighter, just as tasty and even more versatile than other varieties. Lemon is the key ingredient of this creamy soup, perfect to be enjoyed warm.*

# RED LENTIL SOUP

(ZUPPA DI LENTICCHIE ROSSE)

GF-V

*Serves 2–4*

## INGREDIENTS

- 1 onion, cut into strips
- 1 garlic clove, grated
- 250 g (9 oz) red lentils
- 2 dried bay leaves
- warm water, to taste
- 1 parsley sprig
- extra virgin olive oil, to taste
- pinch of sea salt
- 1 dried chilli
- 1 lemon

## METHOD

Heat some oil in a frying pan over low heat. Add the onion and sauté. Add the garlic and stir.

Add the lentils and cook for a few minutes. Add the bay leaves and enough hot water to cover the lentils (add more as it is absorbed).

When the lentils have the desired consistency, remove from the heat. Allow to cool slightly, then blend until you have a creamy texture.

Heat the mixture for 2–4 minutes. Serve hot with crushed red pepper, parsley and a squeeze of lemon.

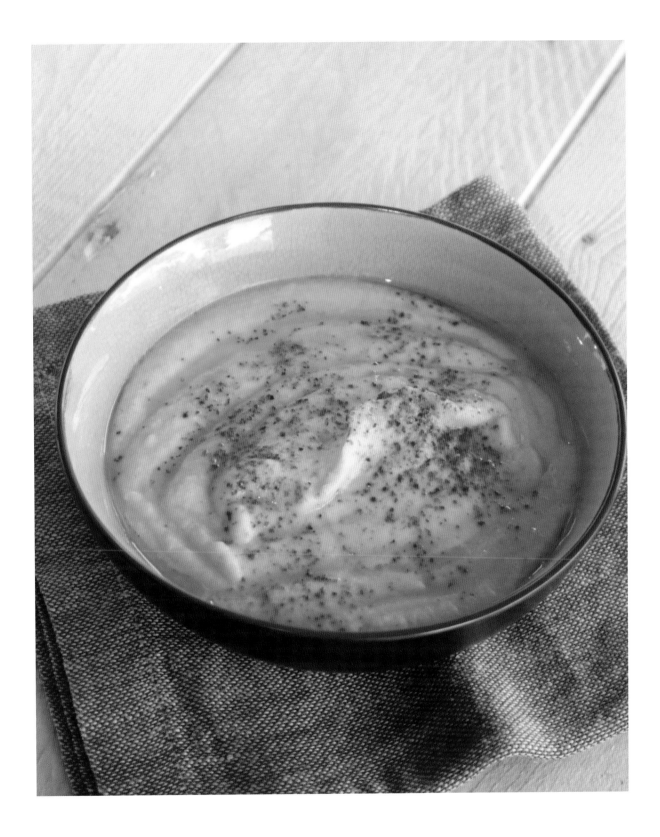

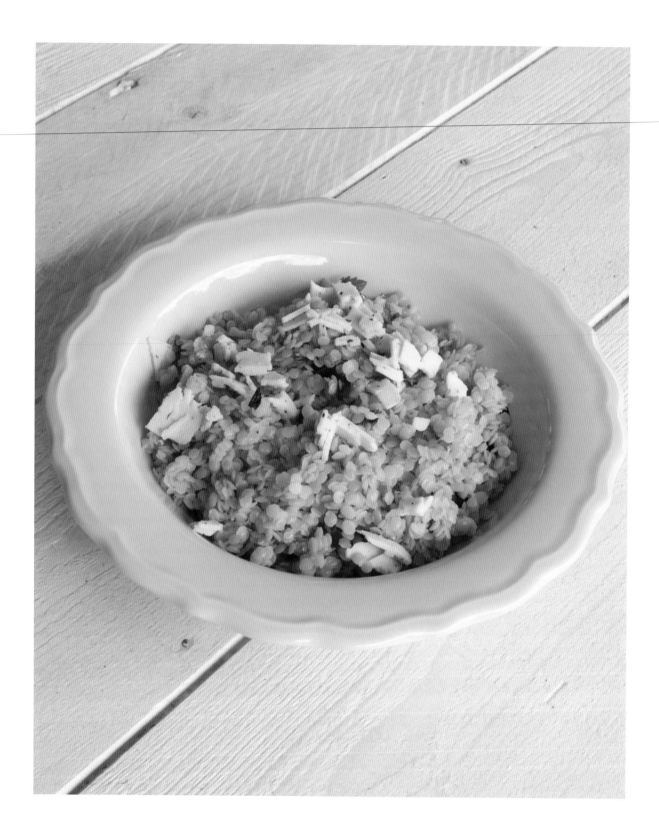

*For people new to vegan cheese, this recipe is an invitation to try it. Fresh and light, vegan cheese is rich in nutrients and is perfect for summer dishes.*

*This recipe is one of my regulars in the hot season. Consumed warm or cold, it is simply delicious.*

# RED LENTILS WITH VEGAN CHEESE

(LENTICCHIE ROSSE CON FORMAGGIO VEGANO)

GF-V

### Serves 2

### INGREDIENTS

- 250 g (9 oz) red lentils
- 1 onion, finely chopped
- 200 g (7 oz) vegan cheese (or goat cheese), cut into cubes
- 1 oregano sprig
- extra virgin olive oil, to taste
- pinch of sea salt
- pepper, to taste

### METHOD

Rinse the red lentils and drain. Add to a saucepan filled with cold water. Bring to the boil over medium heat and cook for 20 minutes, adding salt at the end of cooking.

Heat 4 tablespoons of oil in a frying pan over medium heat. Add the onion and brown. Add the lentils and cook, stirring, for a few minutes for the flavours to combine. Add the vegan cheese and stir to combine.

Place the lentils on a serving dish, add the oregano and extra virgin olive oil and serve.

*Cowpeas are legumes of Asian and African origins. In Italy, they are mainly grown in Veneto, Puglia (Apulia) and Tuscany. They are very nutritious, rich in protein and fibre. This recipe is perfect all year round and is also delicious cold. Ginger gives the freshness and the unmistakable taste. You can also add barley, spelt or rice.*

# SPICY COWPEAS SOUP

(ZUPPA SPEZIATA CON FAGIOLI ALL'OCCHIO)

GF - VEG - V

### Serves 4

**INGREDIENTS**

- 400 g (14 oz) cowpeas
- 1 red onion, sliced
- 1 garlic clove
- 1 carrot, diced
- pinch of sea salt
- white pepper, to taste
- 1 teaspoon ground ginger
- 1 teaspoon chili powder
- 1 tablespoon dry oregano
- extra virgin olive oil, to taste

**METHOD**

Soak the cowpeas with a pinch of baking soda overnight.

The next day, drain the cowpeas and add to a saucepan with the onion, whole garlic, carrot, salt, pepper, ginger and chili powder. Cook the soup over medium heat for about 1 hour 30 minutes to 2 hours, stirring occasionally.

Add the oregano and add a generous dose of extra virgin olive oil. Serve hot, warm or cold, according to taste.

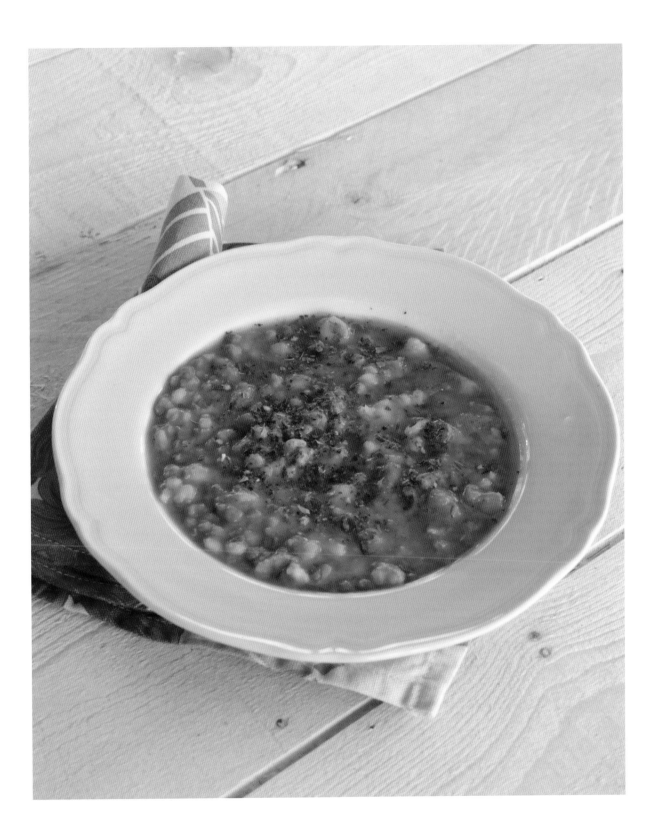

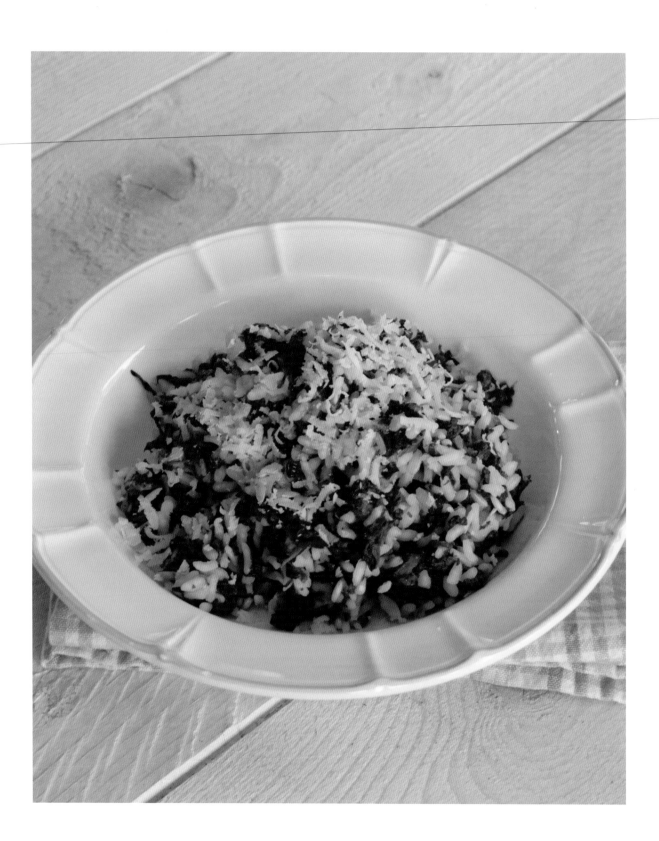

*This recipe has a distinctive flavor, due to an excellent olive oil that highlights the special aroma of the spinach.*

*Simple and quick to prepare, spinach are great on their own, as a snack, accompanied by good rustic bread or as a side dish for eggs, tofu, seitan, in order to have an additional protein, in addition to that found in spinach and Parmigiano.*

# SPINACH WITH PARMIGIANO

(SPINACH CON PARMIGIANO)

V

*Serves 4*

## INGREDIENTS

· 500 g (1 lb 2 oz) baby English spinach
· sea salt, to taste
· extra virgin olive oil, to taste
· 100 g (3$^1/_2$ oz) grated Parmigiano

## METHOD

Put the spinach in a large pot over medium heat and cook for 8–10 minutes. Halfway through cooking, add a pinch of salt.

When cooked, put the spinach in a colander and crush with a spoon to squeeze and remove any remaining water.

Heat the oil in a frying pan over medium heat and add the spinach, 50 g (1$^3/_4$ oz) of the grated Parmigiano and mix.

Serve hot and garnish with the remaining Parmigiano.

*The idea is for a starter but it is also ideal as a main course for an informal brunch in the country.*

# TOFU AND SEITAN SKEWERS

(SPIEDINI DI TOFU E SEITAN)

V

*Serves 4*

## INGREDIENTS

- 3 zucchini (courgettes), sliced
- 3 carrots, sliced
- 6 cherry tomatoes, halved
- 250 g (9 oz) tofu, cut into cubes
- 250 g (9 oz) Seitan, cut into cubes

- extra virgin olive oil, to taste
- 1 handful dry oregano
- pinch of sea salt
- balsamic vinegar, to taste

## METHOD

Blanch the zucchini and carrots in salted water until *al dente*.
Cook the tofu and seitan in a frying pan over medium heat (no oil) for 5 minutes.
Create the skewers with the ingredients available.
In a baking dish, add the oil, oregano, pinch of salt and balsamic vinegar.
Marinate the skewers in the oil mixture for about 1 hour, turning occasionally.

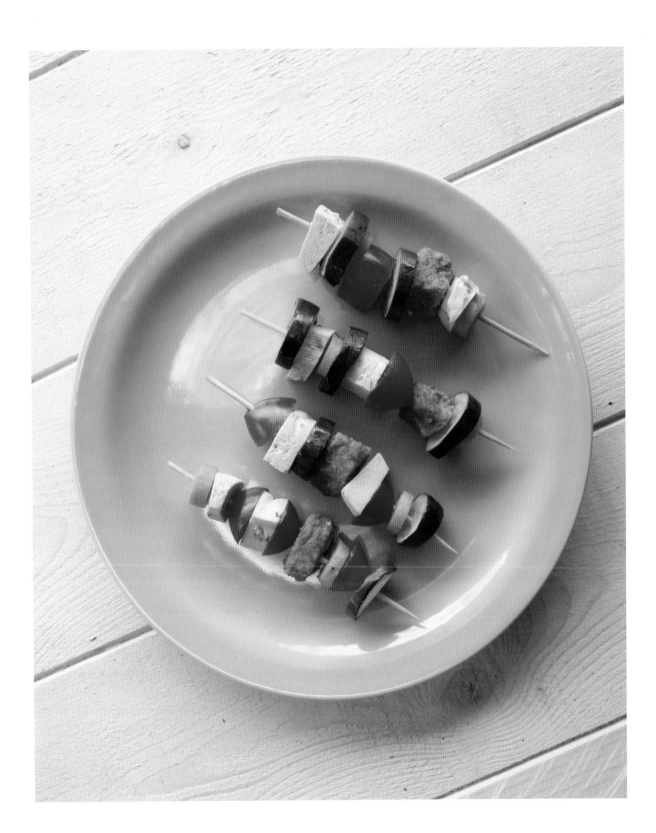

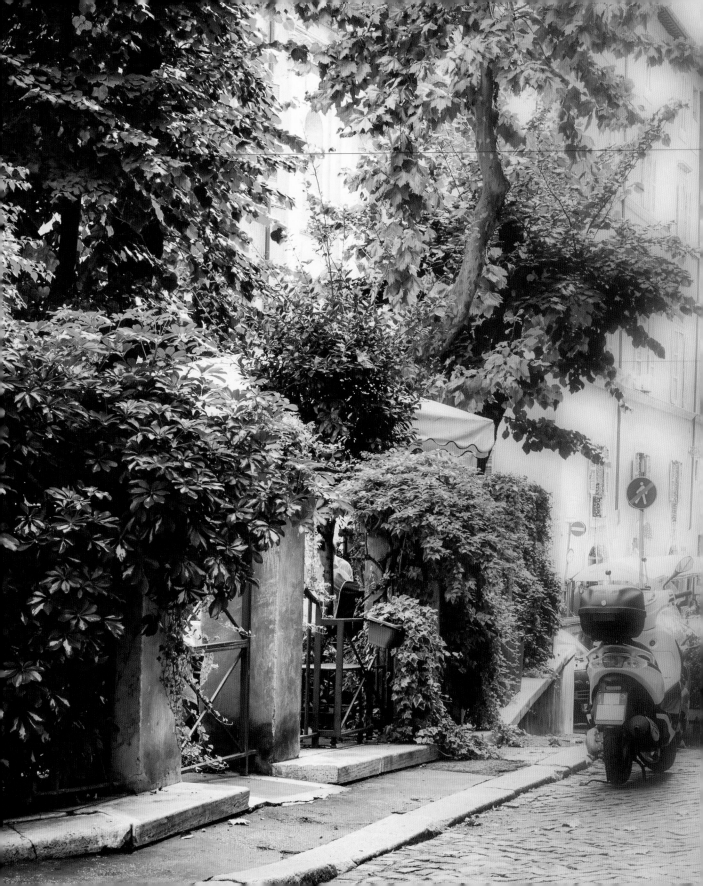

# DESSERTS & SNACKS

I could never give up sweets. I love them. They are a rewarding pause that improves the mood. For this, it is important to use natural sweeteners. They have a low glycemic index and train the palate to appreciate the natural flavours of the food, unlike white sugar which covers the taste of the individual ingredients.

By now, their use is quite common and they can be found in all supermarkets but, for this, we must be careful to choose quality products that are truly natural. For example, not all honey is the same, so it is best to buy organic raw honey, preferably local.

The same applies for raw brown sugar, preferably fairtrade (some industries add molasses to white sugar and sell it as raw sugar).

In this section you will find tips to prepare simple and healthy desserts to enjoy at any time of the day.

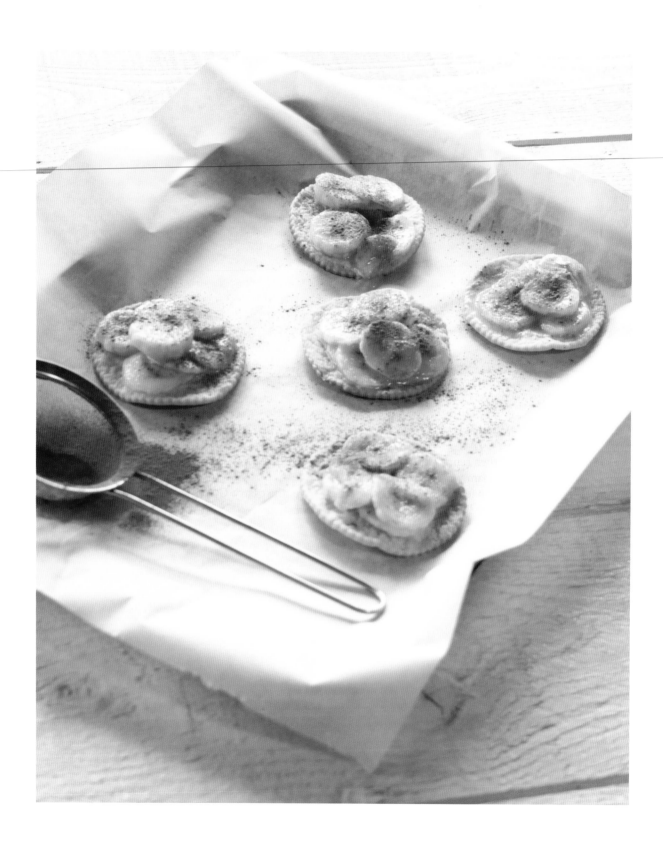

*This recipe is extremely easy and the visual effect is remarkable. In addition, it is perfect at every moment of the day from breakfast, the afternoon snack but also as a light dessert.*

# BANANAS IN SHORTCRUST PASTRY

(SFOGLIATINE DI BANANE)

DF-EF-VEG

## *Serves 4*

### INGREDIENTS

- 250 g (7 oz) organic shortcrust pastry (palm oil free)
- 4 tablespoons sugar-free apricot or peach jam
- juice of 1 lemon
- 3 ripe bananas, sliced
- 1 teaspoon ground cinnamon

### METHOD

Preheat the oven to 180°C (350°F/Gas 4). Line a baking tray with baking paper.

Cut 4 rounds from the shortcrust pastry. Place on the baking tray. Prick the pastry with a fork and cover with baking paper, to avoid swelling.

Bake for 10 minutes, then remove the paper and cook for a further 3 minutes.

Spread the pastry with jam.

Drizzle the bananas with lemon juice. Place the bananas over the pastry. Garnish with a sprinkling of cinnamon. Serve immediately

*These cakes, so delicate and soft, will captivate you. They lend themselves to various uses. Without the chocolate coating, they are perfect for dunking in milk at breakfast or as a snack. With chocolate icing, they are delicious as a dessert.*

# CAKES WITH DRIED APRICOTS AND BANANAS WITH CHOCOLATE GLAZE

(TORTINE DI ALBICOCCHE E BANANE SECCHE CON GLASSA DI CIOCCOLATO)

DF-VEG

*Serves 6-8*

## INGREDIENTS

- 100 g (3$\frac{1}{2}$ oz) pine nuts
- 2 large eggs
- 4 tablespoons extra virgin olive oil (or 100 ml/3$\frac{1}{2}$ fl oz organic cold-pressed
- sunflower oil)
- 4 tablespoons rice milk
- juice and grated zest of 2 red oranges
- 50 g (1$\frac{3}{4}$ oz) raw coconut sugar

- pinch of sea salt
- 300 g (10$\frac{1}{2}$ oz) wholemeal (wholewheat) flour, sifted
- 15 g ($\frac{1}{2}$ oz) organic baking powder
- 50 g (1$\frac{3}{4}$ oz oz) dried apricots (palm oil free)
- 50 g (1$\frac{3}{4}$ oz) raisin (palm oil free)
- 1 handful dried bananas
- 100 g (3$\frac{1}{2}$ oz) dark 85% chocolate

## METHOD

Preheat the oven to 180°C (350°F/Gas 4). Grease eight muffin holes and line with baking paper.

Toast the pine nuts in the oven for 5 minutes. Allow to cool and chop coarsely.

Beat the eggs with the oil, milk, the grated zest of oranges, sugar and pinch of salt.

Add the flour, sifted with baking powder, pine nuts, apricots, roughly chopped, the raisins and the orange juice. Stir to combine.

Pour the mixture into the muffin holes. Add 2–3 dried banana pieces on top and bake for 30 minutes.

Allow to cool, then decorate with melted chocolate.

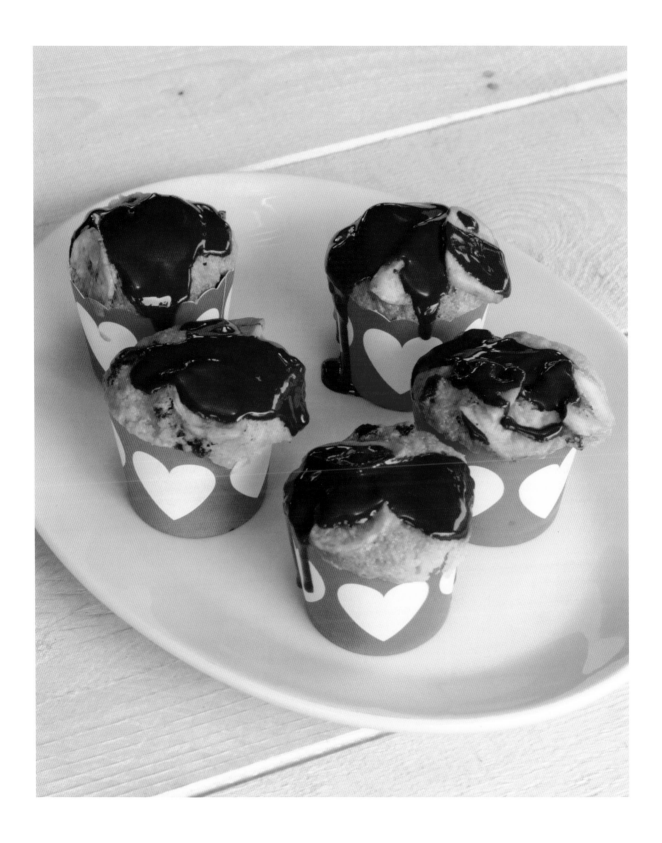

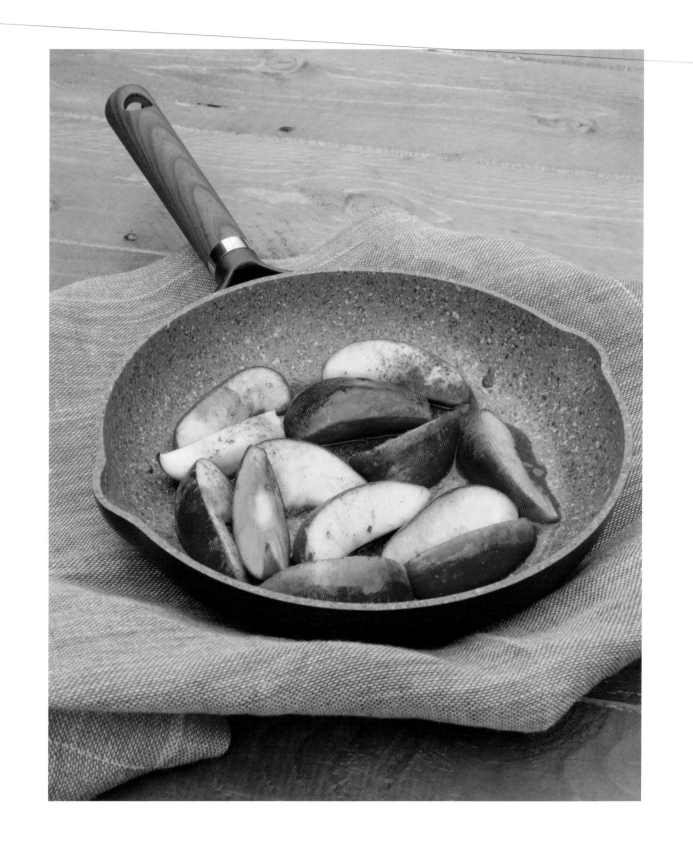

*The crisp and fresh apples are the key ingredient to this recipe.Red apples are perfect for a juicy and tasty dish.*

# CARAMELIZED APPLES

GF

*Serves 2*

## INGREDIENTS

- 2 red apples
- juice of 2 lemons
- 60 g (2¹/₄ oz) raw coconut sugar
- 3 tablespoons water
- 2 teaspoons ground cinnamon

## METHOD

Preheat the oven to 180°C (350°F/Gas 4). Line a baking tray with baking paper.

Wash, dry and cut the apples into slices. Place the apples on the baking tray and sprinkle with the lemon juice.

In a saucepan over medium heat, melt the coconut sugar with the water. Once melted, turn off the heat and add 1 teaspoon cinnamon.

Pour the sugar over the apples, sprinkle with the remaining teaspoon of cinnamon and cook for 10 minutes.

*These small sweets are addictive. Choose a high dark chocolate percentage. The muesli is widely used in Europe. Unlike the granola, muesli (especially if organic), does not contain added oils. Excellent quality muesli will give the required crispness to make special these delights.*

# CHOCOLATE BITES

(CROCCANTINI DI CIOCCOLATO)

V

*Makes about 30*

## INGREDIENTS
· 250 g (9 oz) 80% chopped dark chocolate
· 1 teaspoon organic vanilla bourbon powder
· 200 g (7 oz) organic muesli (or granola, palm oil free)
· 100 g ($3^{1}/_{2}$ oz) puffed brown rice

## METHOD
Melt the chocolate.
Add the vanilla, muesli and puffed brown rice and mix to combine
Pour the mixture into cup cake patty's and refrigerate for 1-2 hours.

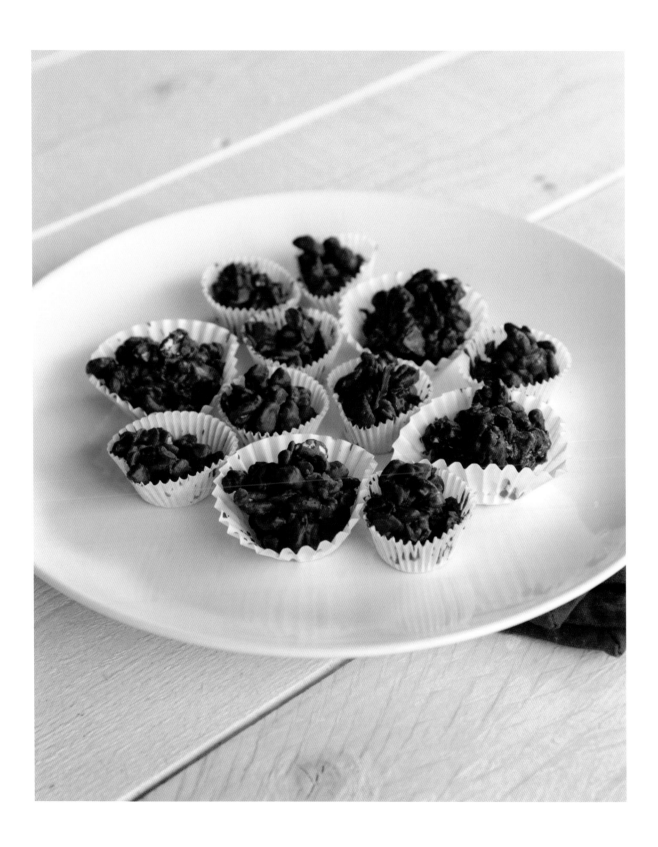

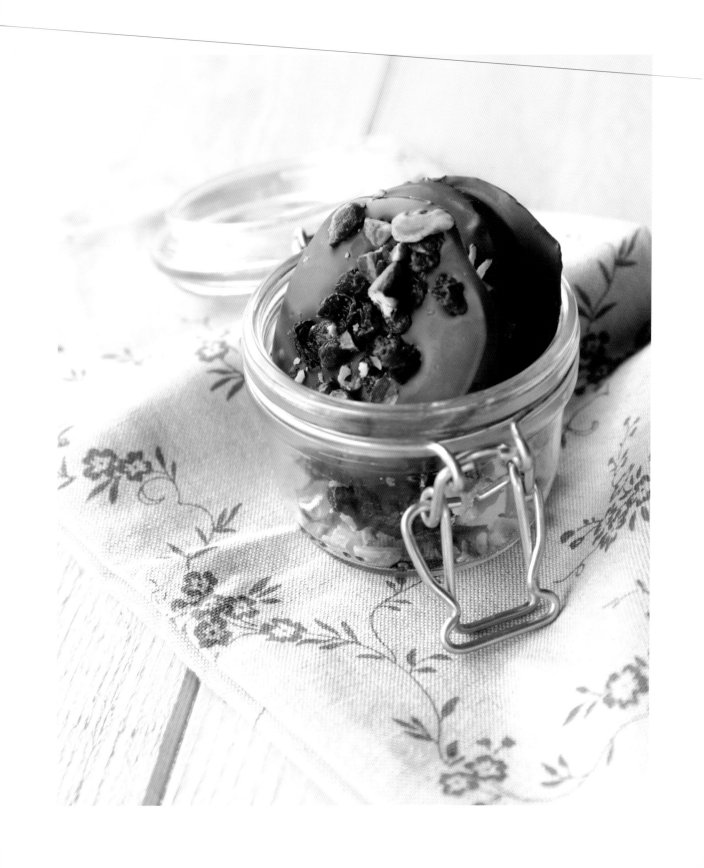

*This is a perfect solution when you do not have many ingredients available and you need something sweet. The final effect is beautiful, like the taste, but only if you use very high quality chocolate.*

# CHOCOLATES WITH DRIED FRUIT

(CIOCCOLATINI CON FRUTTA SECCA)

V

*Makes about 20–25*

**INGREDIENTS**

- 50 g (1³/₄ oz) raisins (palm oil free)
- 1 tablespoon Marsala dessert wine or Rum
- 150 g (5¹/₂ oz) 70% dark chocolate
- 150 g (5¹/₂ oz) 80% dark chocolate
- 50 g (1³/₄ oz) chopped pistachio
- 50 g (1³/₄ oz) chopped walnuts
- 50 g (1³/₄ oz) chopped toasted hazelnuts

**METHOD**

Wash the raisins and soften for 20 minutes in a bowl with warm water. Add a tablespoon of Marsala or Rum. Drain, dry and set aside.

Melt the chocolate, then remove from the heat and allow to cool.

Pour the melted chocolate in spoonfuls on a baking tray lined with baking paper.

Decorate with raisins and the dried fruit. Leave to rest at room temperature until they are solidified. Keep in the fridge.

*These cups are simply delicious. Their velvety texture makes them irresistible. Egg-free and without added sugars, when prepared with milk and rice cream, they become a perfect gluten-free treat, also suitable as a snack.*

# CRUNCHY CHOCOLATE CUPS

(COPPETTE DI CIOCCOLATO CON CROCCANTE)

EF-DF-GF

*Serves 4-6 (it depends on the size of the cups)*

## INGREDIENTS

- 8–10 Medjool dates
- 250 ml (9 fl oz) rice milk
- 2–3 tablespoons cold-pressed organic sunflower oil
- 1 teaspoon ground cinnamon
- pinch of sea salt
- 2 tablespoons brown rice flour
- 200 g (7 oz) 70% chopped dark chocolate
- 60 g (2¼ oz) chopped toasted hazelnuts (or almonds, pistachios, walnuts)

## METHOD

With an immersion blender, blend the dates with 50 ml (1¾ fl oz) rice milk. Add the remaining rice milk, oil, cinnamon, salt and flour. Whisk to combine ingredients.

Bring to the boil and cook for about 5 minutes. Turn off the heat and add the chocolate. Mix well until smooth and shiny.

Pour a layer of chopped hazelnuts on the bottom of the glass. Add the chocolate cream and cover with the other chopped hazelnuts.

Rest the cream at room temperature before serving.

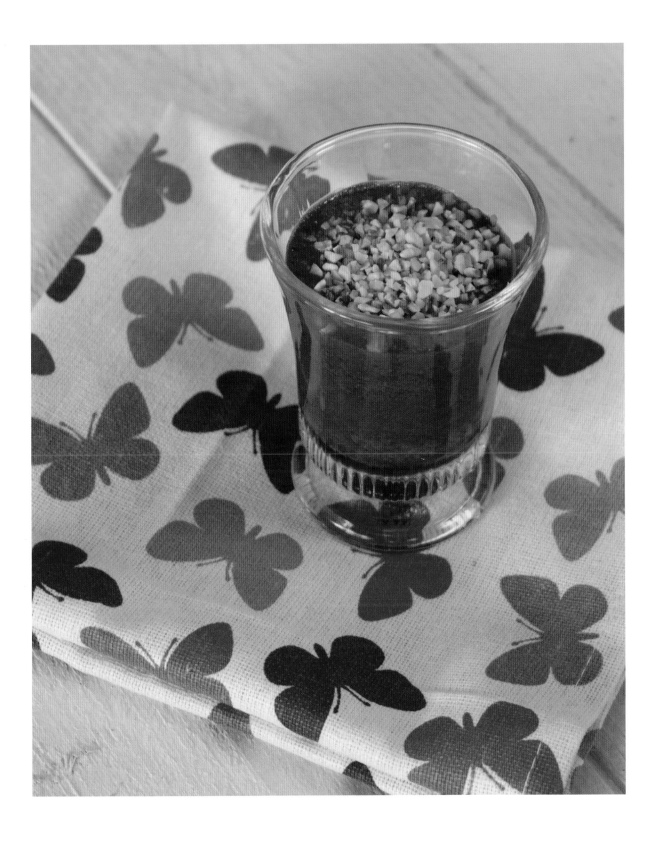

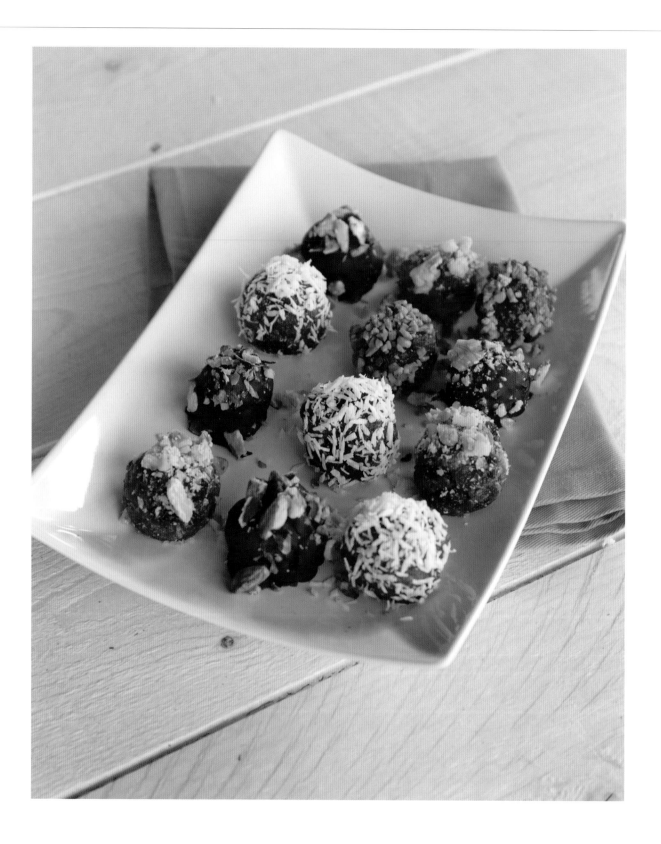

*This is a classic dessert. Dried fruit works wonders and these truffles are a confirmation. My version includes the addition of Sicilian pistachios and the chocolate coating. The Medjool dates are indicated for their softness. Unfortunately, you will not get the same results with other dates.*

# DRIED FRUIT TRUFFLES

(TARTUFI DI FRUTTA SECCA)

EG - GF - VEG

## *Makes about 15 truffles*

### INGREDIENTS

- 80 g (2³/₄ oz) raisins (palm oil free)
- 50 g (1³/₄ oz) dried figs
- 2 tablespoons chopped toasted hazelnuts
- 5 Medjool dates
- 100 g (3¹/₂ oz) 70% dark chocolate

- 1 tablespoon chopped pistachio
- 1 tablespoon chopped toasted hazelnuts (or, almonds, walnuts)
- 1 tablespoon organic coconut flakes

### METHOD

Wash the raisins and soak in warm water. Drain, dry and put in a blender along with the hazelnuts, figs and dates, both chopped.

Blend until you have a smooth dough. Remove a small amount of dough and make small balls. Cool down the balls in the fridge.

Melt chocolate in a double boiler. Allow to cool.

Dip the balls in chocolate. Garnish with the pistachio, hazelnuts, coconut flakes and/or other dried fruit. Allow the chocolate to thicken at room temperature and store the truffles in the refrigerator until ready to serve.

*This is one of the dessert cakes prepared by my mother that I love most. She has always replaced the white sugar with raw honey. Delicious. My version with coconut sugar is just as satisfying and gives an even more distinctive flavour.*

# PISTACHIO AND LIMONCELLO CAKE

(TORTA DI PISTACCHIO E LIMONCELLO)

GF-V

*Serves 8–10*

## INGREDIENTS

- 200 g (7 oz) pistachios
- 100 g (3¹/₂ oz) toasted hazelnuts
- 80 g (2³/₄ oz) raw coconut sugar
- zest of 1 lemon
- 2 carrots, chopped
- 1 egg
- pinch of sea salt

- 1 teaspoon organic vanilla bourbon powder
- 100 g (3¹/₂ oz) brown rice flour, sifted
- 15 g (¹/₂ oz) organic baking powder

### Topping
- 200 g (7 oz) high-quality white chocolate
- 1 tablespoon limoncello

## METHOD

Preheat the oven to 180°C (350°F/Gas 4). Line a 35cm round baking tin with baking paper.

Process the pistachios in a food processor with the hazelnuts, coconut sugar and lemon zest. Pour into a bowl. Blend the carrots with the eggs salt and vanilla. Add this mixture to the pistachio and hazelnut flours. Combine the brown rice flour, baking powder and mix well with each other all the ingredients.

Bake for 35-40 minutes.

Melt the white chocolate in a double boiler. Remove from the heat and add the tablespoon limoncello. Once the cake has cooled, decorate with the melted chocolate. Leave to rest at room temperature for 10–15 minutes before serving.

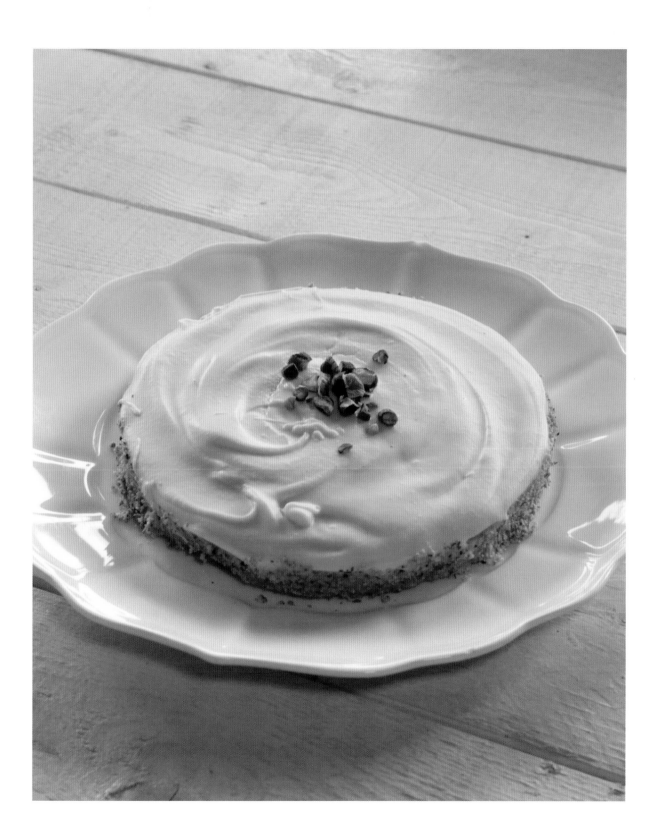

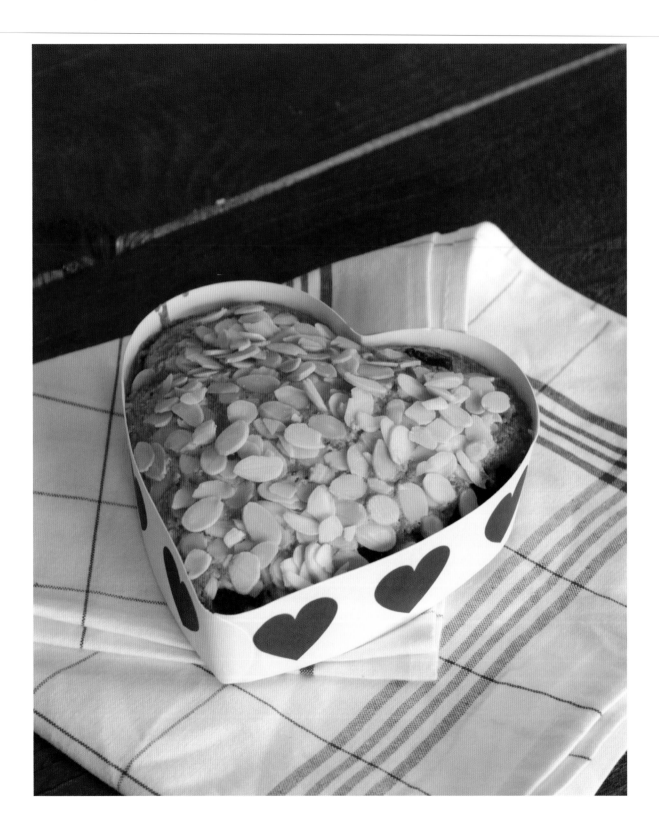

*I love to serve this cake with ice cream when raspberries are in season. They give a delicate flavour to these small cakes and make them a very soft dough. I also like to add dried cranberries, when available, not only for the taste but also because, in Italy, they are not easy to find, and, like all rare food, they become a precious ingredient.*

*These cakes are perfect as dessert for an informal brunch or lunch.*

*Raspberry and almond cakes*

# RASPBERRY AND ALMOND CAKE

(TORTINE DI LAMPONI E MANDORLE)

V

*Serves 6-8*

## INGREDIENTS

- 4 tablespoons extra virgin olive oil or 100 ml (3¹⁄₂ fl oz) organic cold-pressed sunflower oil
- 100 g (3¹⁄₂ oz) raw coconut sugar
- 50 ml (1³⁄₄ fl oz) rice milk
- 2 eggs
- 300 g (10¹⁄₂ oz) wholemeal (whole-wheat) flour, sifted
- 15 g (¹⁄₂ oz) organic baking powder
- 50 g (1³⁄₄ oz) toasted chopped almonds
- zest of 1 lemon
- pinch of sea salt
- 100 g (3¹⁄₂ oz) fresh raspberries
- 80 g (2³⁄₄ oz) dried cranberries (palm oil free)
- 100 g (3¹⁄₂ oz) sliced almonds

## METHOD

Preheat the oven to 180°C (350°F/Gas 4). Lightly grease eight muffin holes.

Mix the oil and sugar. Add the milk, egg yolks, flour, baking powder, almonds, lemon zest, a pinch of salt and mix with an electric mixer.

Stir in the egg whites, raspberries and cranberries.

Pour the mixture into the muffin holes. Cover with the sliced almonds and bake for 40 minutes. Allow to cool in the tin for 5 minutes before turning out onto a wire rack to cool completely.

*A colourful and tasty snack which can be eaten for breakfast or any time of the day.*
*Fresh seasonal fruit, preferably organic, is the basic ingredient to ensure a unique flavor.*
*You can replace the honey with the syrup of dates and ginger with vanilla or cinnamon.*

# SUMMER TART

(SFOGLIA ESTIVA)

VEG - DF

*Serves 4–6*

## INGREDIENTS

· 10 apricots, halved
· 15 strawberries, halved
· 1 tablespoon raw honey
· juice of 1 lemon
· 1 teaspoon ground ginger
· 2 tablespoons organic sugar-free apricot or strawberry jam
· 250 g (9 oz) organic wholemeal (whole-wheat) puff pastry (palm oil free)
· 1 handful mint leaves

## METHOD

Preheat the oven to 180°C (350°F/Gas 4). Lightly grease a 35 cm round baking tray.

Place the fruit in a saucepan. Add a heaping tablespoon of honey and the lemon juice and cook for 5 minutes. Remove from the heat, add the ginger and stir.

Roll out the pastry and spread with the jam. Add the fruit.

Bake for 15 minutes. Serve immediately.

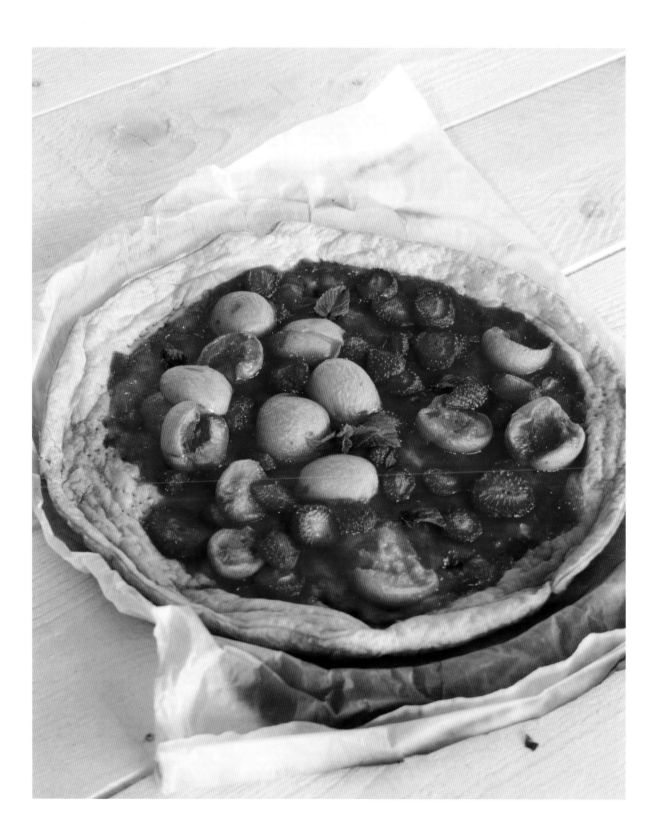

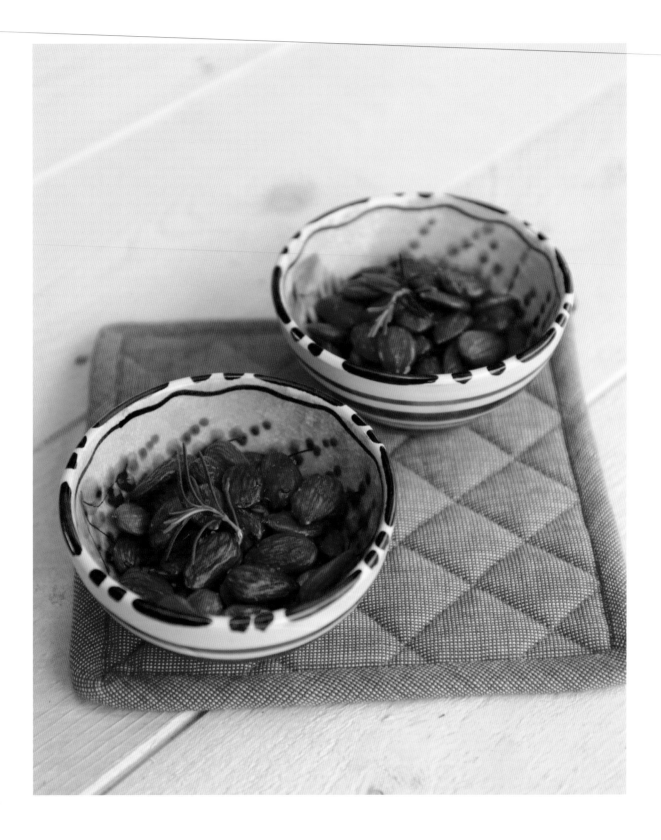

*I know, it is not a 'recipe' but for us Italians, recipes are not those that require cooking or long preparation methods. For us, a recipe is also assembled with a few high-quality ingredients.*

*Sicilian almonds are one of those Italian culinary specialties that must be tried at least once in life. A little salt, rosemary, excellent olive oil and it's done.*

# TOASTED ALMONDS WITH ROSEMARY

(MANDORLE TOSTATE CON ROSMARINO)

GF-V

*Serves 2*

**INGREDIENTS**

· 100 g (3½ oz) whole almonds
· pinch of sea salt
· 1 rosemary sprig
· extra virgin olive oil, to taste

**METHOD**

Toast the almonds in the oven for 10 minutes at 180°C (350°F/Gas 4).

Once toasted, allow to cool, put them in a bowl and season with a pinch of salt, finely chopped rosemary and olive oil.

Serve immediately.

*This is one of my favourite afternoon snacks. These cups, with their high nutritional value provided by dried fruit and seeds, are still best suited for breakfast.*

# YOGHURT AND GRANOLA CUPS

(COPPETTE DI YOGURT E GRANOLA)

V

*Serves 8–10 small cups*

## INGREDIENTS

- 150 g (5$^1$/$_2$ oz) oatmeal flakes
- 100 g (3$^1$/$_2$ oz) chopped toasted hazelnuts
- 50 g (1$^3$/$_4$ oz) chopped toasted almonds
- 1 tablespoon pumpkin seeds
- 1 tablespoon toasted sesame seeds
- 2 tablespoons ground cinnamon

- 4 tablespoons organic cold-pressed sunflower oil
- 2 tablespoons date nectar
- 50 g (1$^3$/$_4$ oz) raisins
- 50 g (1$^3$/$_4$ oz) chopped dried bananas, palm oil free
- 250 g (9 oz) sugar-free rice (or soy) yoghurt

## METHOD

Preheat the oven to 200°C (400°F/Gas 6). Line a baking try with baking paper.

Combine the oatmeal flakes, hazelnuts, almonds, pumpkin seeds and sesame in a bowl. Add the cinnamon, oil, date nectar and mix.

Spread the granola on the baking tray and bake for 15–20 minutes, stirring occasionally.

Pour the granola in a bowl, add the raisins, dried bananas and mix.

On the bottom of each glass add the granola, then a spoonful of yoghurt and cover with more granola and dried bananas.

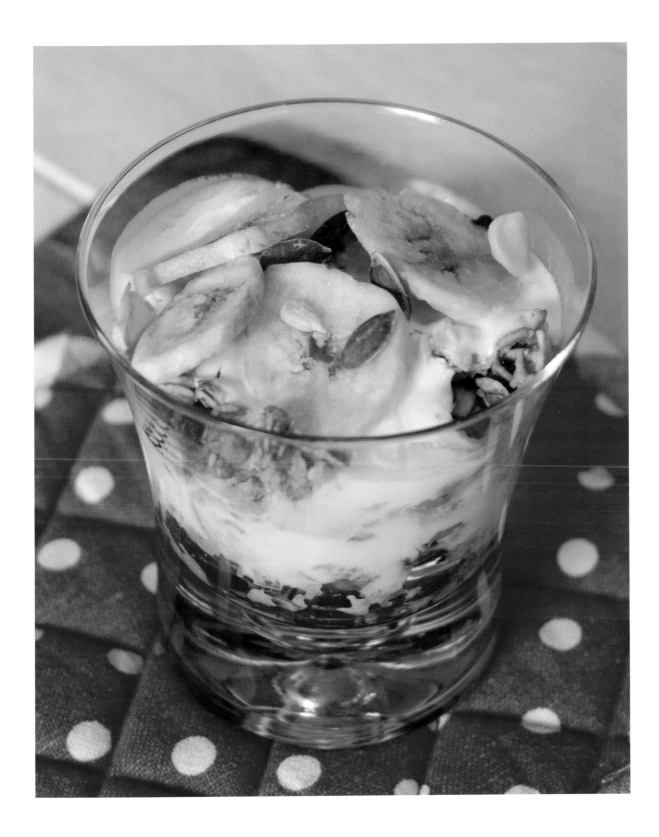

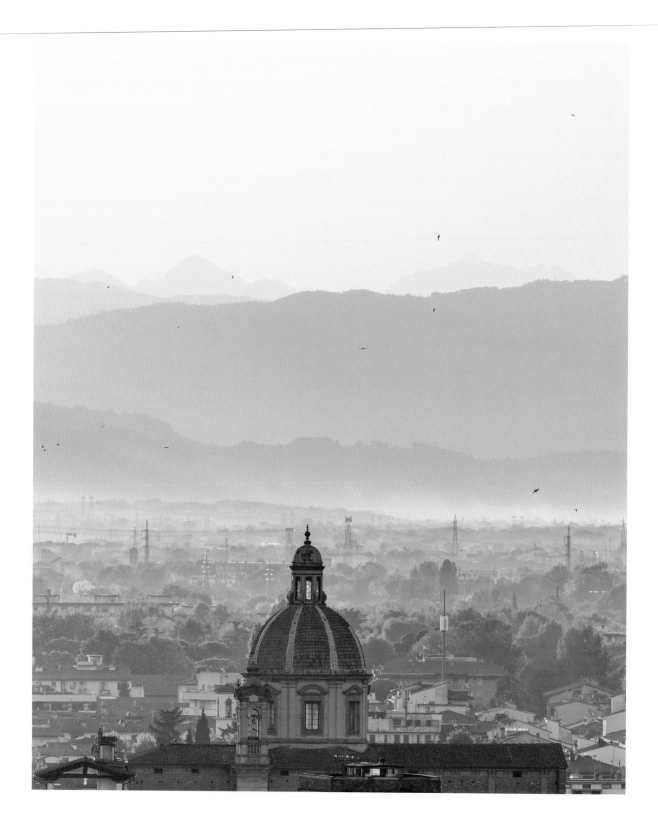

# ACKNOWLEDGEMENTS

Many thanks to:

Fiona Shultz, Monique Butterworth, Christine King, Gordana Trifunovic, Andrew Quinlan, James Mills-Hicks and all New Holland Publishers team for always believing in my work with enthusiasm and to create stunning books; and a special thanks to Jessica Nelson for the excellent editing.

As always, to my family for everything.

To my super tester crew: Piero Pardini, who always enthusiastically supports my every publishing project; Alfio Scuderi who had the inspiration for the beautiful title; Giuseppe Giustolisi for the wonderful photos that highlight each of my recipe.

# INDEX

**VEGETARIAN AND VEGAN PROTEINS**

**DESSERTS & SNACKS**

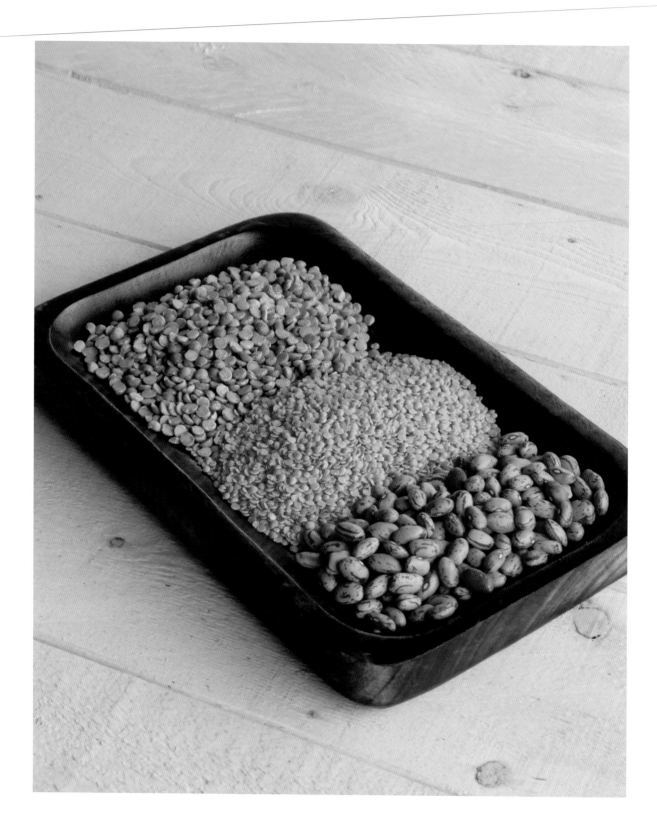

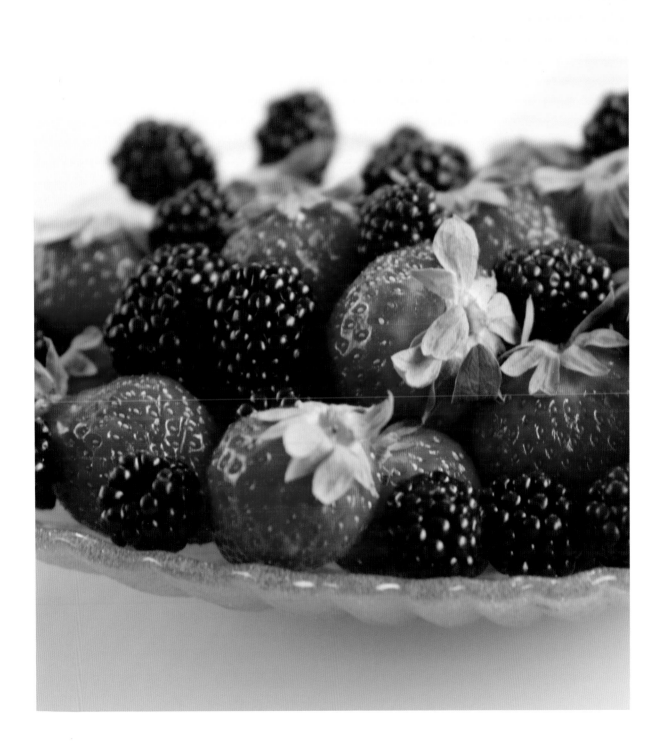